Fibromyalgia

Dawn A. Marcus · Atul Deodhar

Fibromyalgia

A Practical Clinical Guide

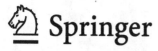 Springer

Dawn A. Marcus
Department of Anesthesiology
University of Pittsburgh
3550 Terrace St.
A-1305 Scaife Hall
Pittsburgh, PA 15261, USA
dawnpainmd@yahoo.com

Atul Deodhar, MD
Division of Arthritis & Rheumatic
  Diseases (OP09)
Oregon Health & Science University
3181 SW Sam Jackson Park Road
Portland, OR 97239, USA
deodhara@ohsu.edu

Additional material to this book can be downloaded from http://extras.springer.com

ISBN 978-1-4419-1608-2   e-ISBN 978-1-4419-1609-9
DOI 10.1007/978-1-4419-1609-9
Springer New York Dordrecht Heidelberg London

Library of Congress Control Number: 2010932233

Printed on acid-free paper

Springer is part of Springer Science+Business Media (www.springer.com)

Preface

Fibromyalgia affects about 2–3% of adults worldwide, with women affected three to six times as often as men. While fibromyalgia is a chronic pain disorder, patients with fibromyalgia typically present with a complicated constellation of painful and non-painful complaints, including disabling fatigue, sleep disturbance, and neuropsychological symptoms. Anxiety, mental distress, and cognitive dysfunction are reported by nearly two in every three fibromyalgia patients. One in three fibromyalgia sufferers reports current depression, with a history of depression in over half. Headaches are also common. Evaluating fibromyalgia patients requires an understanding of the complex nature of this condition and the myriad of likely fibromyalgia-related complaints.

Fibromyalgia is often poorly understood and unrecognized. Failure to identify and treat fibromyalgia patients effectively can lead patients to feel misunderstood, confused, and frustrated that their symptoms are not believed by their healthcare providers, and discouraged about leading a full and rewarding life. Fibromyalgia typically affects adults during what should be fulfilling and productive years, when they are caring for families, developing careers, and making a strong impact on their communities. The good news for our patients is that fibromyalgia is straightforward to diagnose, with symptoms effectively reduced using a wide range of proven medication, non-medication, and non-traditional treatments.

> When I told a friend who is also a fibromyalgia patient about this new book, she responded, *When I was diagnosed with fibromyalgia almost 10 years ago, there wasn't as much information as there has been in the last few years. I'm glad to see that the medical community is finally recognizing this condition and treating fibromyalgia more seriously and with more compassion.*

Fibromyalgia: A Practical Clinical Guide consolidates years of experience in identifying and treating fibromyalgia from pain management and rheumatology perspectives. The authors' wealth of clinical practice and research has been combined to provide easy-to-understand and practical tips for clinicians caring for

fibromyalgia patients. Case presentations and quotations from active fibromyalgia patients help highlight complaints and concerns commonly experienced by
fibromyalgia sufferers. Dr. Dawn A. Marcus is a neurologist, pain management specialist, and professor at the University of Pittsburgh, with expertise treating and
researching fibromyalgia. She is an active writer and lecturer on topics related
to chronic pain and fibromyalgia and has authored several practical books for
both healthcare providers and lay audiences. Dr. Atul Deodhar is a rheumatologist, associate professor of medicine at the Oregon Health and Science University,
and director of Rheumatology Clinics at Oregon Health and Science University.
Drs. Marcus and Deodhar previously collaborated to produce *Chronic Pain: An
Atlas of Investigation and Management.*

Fibromyalgia: A Practical Clinical Guide is designed to cut through the
hype about fibromyalgia and provide clinicians with up-to-date information about
fibromyalgia pathogenesis and clinical evaluation, as well as evidence-based guidelines for effective treatment. This book includes fully referenced, cutting-edge
information on this fast-growing field and provides practical pointers for effectively managing fibromyalgia patients. Treatment recommendations focus on targeting symptoms most likely to respond to therapy and prescribing medication,
non-medication, and alternative/complementary treatments that have been proven
to reduce fibromyalgia symptoms. Boxes, tables, and figures are used widely
throughout the text to provide quick reference for the busy clinician seeking information. Clinically proven tools to help evaluate and treat fibromyalgia patients
include handouts for recording and monitoring fibromyalgia symptoms and severity, exercise instructions, and self-help guides for psychological pain management
techniques. Additional materials may be accessed through Dr. Marcus' Web site
www.dawnmarcusmd.com. Both authors are eager to receive comments and suggestions for additions and improvements to the book through a link available at this
Web site.

Pittsburgh, Pennsylvania   Dawn A. Marcus
Portland, Oregon   Atul Deodhar

Contents

Part I
Background

Introduction

Key Chapter Points

- Fibromyalgia-like symptoms were first discussed in the 1800s.
- The American College of Rheumatology published classification criteria for a unique and specific syndrome of fibromyalgia in 1990.
- Today's fibromyalgia should not be confused with previously identified vague and non-specific syndrome diagnoses, like muscular rheumatism and fibrositis.
- Fibromyalgia sufferers are very interested in having healthcare providers who take their complaints seriously and treat them as credible patients.
- Fibromyalgia patients need to receive a diagnosis from their doctors that does not imply their symptoms are entirely explained by stress or psychological distress.

Keywords Classification · Credibility · Diagnosis · Fibrositis · Muscular rheumatism

Fibromyalgia patients endorse a plethora of physical and psychological symptoms that they generally attribute to their diagnosis of fibromyalgia (Table 1) [1]. The wide range of seemingly unrelated symptoms has led many healthcare providers to view fibromyalgia complaints with skepticism. Healthcare providers may wonder if patients can truly experience such a wide mixture of symptoms or if these reports are embellished or exaggerated when they contrast with the seemingly unremarkable general physical examination that characteristically accompanies the diagnosis of fibromyalgia.

Fibromyalgia is a relatively new diagnosis that continues to be shrouded in controversy, skepticism, and misperceptions within the healthcare community [2]. Today's diagnosis of fibromyalgia has been described by various terms throughout history (Box 1) [3]. A consolation of symptoms including aches, pain, stiffness, sleep disturbance, and fatigue had long been termed *muscular rheumatism* to differentiate symptoms from those caused by joint disease. As doctors evaluated patients with muscular rheumatism, they began to describe tender points and nodules, generally attributing these to an inflammatory disorder and muscle pathology. In 1904, Sir William Gowers introduced the term *fibrositis* to describe what he believed were

D.A. Marcus, A. Deodhar, *Fibromyalgia*, DOI 10.1007/978-1-4419-1609-9_1,
© Springer Science+Business Media, LLC 2011

Table 1 Symptoms endorsed by fibromyalgia patients (based on van Ittersum [1])

Symptom category	Patients experiencing symptom (%)	Patients attributing symptom to fibromyalgia[a] (%)
Constitutional		
Fatigue	94	95
Weight loss	15	12
Sleep difficulties	68	62
Neurological		
Pain	92	90
Headaches	54	32
Dizziness	44	29
Musculoskeletal		
Stiff joints	87	85
Weakness	78	82
Gastrointestinal		
Stomach upset	63	46
Nausea	25	12
Respiratory		
Breathlessness	31	11
Wheezing	21	16
Other		
Sore eyes	52	25
Sore throat	21	6

[a]Most participants only answered the question about symptom attribution to fibromyalgia if they experienced the symptom in question; in some cases, however, fibromyalgia participants not experiencing a symptom reported that they believed that symptom would be attributed to fibromyalgia if it occurred. For this reason, more people attributed fatigue and weakness to fibromyalgia than actually were experiencing those symptoms.

Box 1 History of Fibromyalgia (Based on Inanici [3])

- *Muscular rheumatism* used to describe non-joint-related generalized pain and constitutional symptoms in the 1800s.
- Neurologist Beard introduced the term *neurasthenia* to describe generalized pain and constitutional symptoms as the result of physiological impact from psychological stress in 1880.
- Gowers coined the phrase *fibrositis* to denote inflammatory nature of rheumatism in 1904.
- Terms *myofascitis, myofibrositis, and neurofibrositis* suggested by Albee in 1927, Murray in 1929, and Clayton in 1930, respectively.
- *Interstitial myofibrositis* suggested by Awad in 1973.
- *Fibromyalgia* coined in 1976 by Hench.
- Fibromyalgia confirmed as a unique symptom constellation in a controlled study by Yunus and colleagues in 1981.
- American College of Rheumatology established classification criteria for fibromyalgia.

tender areas of inflammation in patients with rheumatism, although tissue studies performed later failed to identify inflammatory changes [4]. In the early 1970s, Smythe and Moldofsky helped to validate the credibility of fibrositis by noting the consistency of symptoms, tender point locations, and sleep dysfunction [5, 6]. The term *fibromyalgia* was introduced in 1976, denoting an understanding that symptoms were not inflammatory in nature. Yunus and colleagues published the first controlled study evaluating symptoms in 50 patients diagnosed with fibromyalgia and 50 controls in 1981, confirming the anecdotal impression that fibromyalgia included a constellation of symptoms that are now accepted as typical of fibromyalgia, including tender points, pain, sleep disturbance, and gastrointestinal disturbance [7]. The American College of Rheumatology later published clinical classification criteria in 1990 [8].

Practical pointer

Classification criteria for fibromyalgia were published in 1990.

Establishing classification criteria allowed consistent communication among clinicians and researchers that fueled an interest in epidemiological, pathophysiological, and treatment studies. Lack of confirmatory diagnostic data from laboratory or radiographic measures, however, has impeded research and allowed continued skepticism about the validity of fibromyalgia as a unique medical syndrome. The low regard given to fibromyalgia by medical providers was highlighted in a recent study that asked general practitioners to rank 38 common medical conditions, based on each condition's prestige within the medical community [9]. Each condition was rated using a scale from 1 (low prestige) to 9 (high prestige), with an average score among all diseases calculated at 5.1. The top ranking conditions were, in descending order: myocardial infarction, leukemia, spleen rupture, brain tumor, pulmonary embolism, testicular cancer, and angina, with scores ranging from 7.2 to 6.5. Fibromyalgia ranked at the very bottom of the list, with a prestige score of only 2.3. Fibromyalgia was the only medical condition to receive an average score below 3. Rankings by senior physicians and students yielded similar results, with fibromyalgia consistently taking the lowest position.

Practical pointer

Among common medical conditions, doctors rank fibromyalgia with the lowest stature.

Case presentation

Sheryl S. is a 34-year-old wife, mother, and publications director for a university. She's also a fibromyalgia patient. "What doctors should do is listen to their patients – really listen. We fibromyalgia patients need our doctors to understand how disruptive our symptoms are to our lives and treat our complaints seriously. I've had some doctors suggest that I'm complaining because my life isn't full enough. I have a wonderful family, am very active in my Church, and have an exciting career at a growing university. My fibromyalgia symptoms are real, disruptive, and not a substitute for something that's missing in my life!"

Although healthcare providers may not feel fibromyalgia is an important condition, the prevalence of fibromyalgia and its association with substantial disability (as described in the chapter "Fibromyalgia Definition and Epidemiology") necessitate actively addressing this syndrome with affected patients. In a poignant report of interviews of patients with fibromyalgia about their needs for healthcare, patients focused on the need to receive a diagnosis from their doctors that did not imply their symptoms were psychologically based (Box 2) [10]. There was a strong focus on feeling believed by their doctors, with reports of "no objective findings" leading patients to feeling mistrusted. Patients need to know that their doctors believe fibromyalgia is a valid condition, understand the nature and causes of fibromyalgia, and will offer necessary treatment advice to adequately address fibromyalgia symptoms.

Box 2 Important aspects of clinical care for fibromyalgia patients (based on Haugli [10])

- Receive a somatic diagnosis.
- Understand their doctors believe them and treat their complaints seriously.
- Receive an explanation about the causes or physiological basis of fibromyalgia symptoms.
- Understand why specific treatments are being recommended.
- Receive information about managing specific symptoms.
- Have a clinical environment that is open to the patients asking questions.

Summary

- Fibromyalgia has been used as a diagnosis for only about 35 years, with classification criteria established in 1990.
- Older terms, like *muscular rheumatism* and *fibrositis*, were used to describe vague and poorly understood chronic pain syndromes.
- The diagnosis of *fibromyalgia* refers to a unique chronic pain syndrome, defined by the American College of Rheumatology classification criteria in 1990.
- Because of the diverse constellation of symptoms experienced by fibromyalgia patients and the lack of objective abnormalities on standard clinical laboratory and radiographic testing, skepticism about the validity of fibromyalgia has persisted.
- Fibromyalgia patients need to understand their healthcare providers believe their reports are credible. Patients should also be told when their diverse symptoms are characteristic of typical fibromyalgia symptoms.
- Effective care of fibromyalgia patients requires healthcare providers to have a full understanding of fibromyalgia: its diagnosis, what is known about its pathophysiology, and strategies for reducing important patient symptoms.

References

1. Van Ittersum MW, van Wilgen CP, Hilberdink WA, Groothoff JW, van der Schans CP. Illness perceptions in patients with fibromyalgia. Patient Educ Couns. 2009;74:53–60.
2. Wolfe F. Fibromyalgia wars. J Rheumatol. 2009;36:671–8.
3. Inanici F, Yunus MB. History of fibromyalgia: past to present. Curr Pain Headache Rep. 2004;8:369–78.
4. Gowers WR. Lumbago: its lessons and analogues. BMJ. 1904;i:117–21.
5. Smythe H. Nonarticular rheumatism and psychogenic musculoskeletal syndromes. In: McCarty DJ, editors. Arthritis and allied conditions. 8th ed. Philadelphia: Lea & Febiger; 1972. pp. 881–91.
6. Moldofsky H, Scarisbrick P, England R, Smythe H. Musculoskeletal symptoms and non-REM sleep disturbance in patients with "fibrositis syndrome" and healthy subjects. Psychosom Med. 1975;37:341–51.
7. Yunus M, Masi AT, Calabro JJ, Miller KA, Feigenbaum SL. Primary fibromyalgia (fibrositis): clinical study of 50 patients with matched normal controls. Semin Arthritis Rheum. 1981;11:151–71.
8. Wolfe F, Smythe HA, Yunus MB, et al. The American College of Rheumatology 1990 Criteria for the Classification of Fibromyalgia. Report of the Multicenter Criteria Committee. Arthritis Rheum. 1990;33:160–72.
9. Album D, Estin S. Do diseases have a prestige hierarchy? A survey among physicians and medical students. Soc Sci Med. 2008;66:182–8.
10. Haugli L, Strand E, Finset A. How do patients with rheumatic disease experience their relationship with their doctors? A qualitative study of experiences of stress and support in the doctor-patient relationship. Patient Educ Couns. 2004;52:169–74.

Fibromyalgia Definition and Epidemiology

Key Chapter Points

- Fibromyalgia is a chronic, painful condition characterized by widespread pain and positive tender points on physical examination.
- Fibromyalgia affects about 2–3% of adults worldwide, although prevalence is lower in Asia.
- Women are more likely to have fibromyalgia than men.
- Fibromyalgia is co-morbid with other rheumatologic conditions, headaches, chronic fatigue syndrome, irritable bowel syndrome, depression, and anxiety.
- Patients with fibromyalgia experience substantial disability, healthcare utilization, and disease-related costs.

Keywords Co-morbidity · Cost · Disability · Gender · Prevalence

Fibromyalgia is recognized as a condition resulting in both chronic, widespread pain and a variety of somatic complaints. The symptoms reported by fibromyalgia patients often contrast sharply with their characteristically unremarkable musculoskeletal and neurological examinations, with normal laboratory and radiographic tests. Despite normal physical examinations and testing, however, fibromyalgia patients are typically afflicted with substantial disability and emotional distress.

> **Case:** Lynn S. was diagnosed with fibromyalgia at age 32. Symptoms began shortly after the delivery of her son that was complicated by prolonged labor and a post-delivery incision infection. "After my son was born, I noticed that it was harder and harder for me to do things I would normally do. I was in pain all the time, fatigued, yet suffering insomnia symptoms. I went through a year and a half of not knowing what was wrong, thinking I was crazy and must be imagining this stuff. I had a bone scan, carpal tunnel test for numbness in my wrists, and a host of other tests that turned up nothing. My doctors kept telling me my symptoms were caused by my busy schedule as a young mother,

D.A. Marcus, A. Deodhar, *Fibromyalgia*, DOI 10.1007/978-1-4419-1609-9_2,
© Springer Science+Business Media, LLC 2011

working full time, and being very active with community groups. I found this offensive – I was young and I didn't think what I was doing was so over the top. . .it was normal. The doctors seemed to be suggesting that I was the cause for my symptoms, and I knew the way I was feeling wasn't my fault. Finally, a resident at my family doctor's office suggested I see a rheumatologist where I was diagnosed with fibromyalgia. I had no idea at the time what fibromyalgia was, but I would certainly find out in the ensuing months and years!"

Defining Fibromyalgia

Fibromyalgia is a diffuse, chronic pain associated with tender body areas and somatic complaints. Fibromyalgia pain is widespread, although the areas affected by pain often fluctuate, with different areas perceived as more or less problematic on different days. By definition, patients with exclusively localized or focal pain complaints will not be diagnosed with fibromyalgia. A diagnosis of fibromyalgia requires a patient's description of widespread pain, along with the presence of at least 11 of 18 possible tender points (Box 1). Tender points are 18 predetermined areas that tend to be painful with pressure in patients with fibromyalgia. A complete description of tender points is provided in the chapter "Assessment and Diagnosis."

Practical pointer

Fibromyalgia is a widespread, chronic pain condition with at least 11 positive tender points on physical examination.

Box 1 Diagnosis of Fibromyalgia (Based on American College of Rheumatology Criteria; Wolfe [1])

- Widespread body pain
  - Pain on both left and right sides of the body
  - Pain above and below the waist
  - Axial pain present
- Pain persisting ≥3 months
- ≥11 of 18 tender points painful to 4 kg pressure

Most patients with fibromyalgia experience a wide variety of fluctuating symptoms in addition to body pain [1]. The diversity of fibromyalgia symptoms was highlighted in the results of a survey of 2,569 fibromyalgia sufferers visiting the National Fibromyalgia Association Web site [2]. Most of the respondents were female (97%) with a mean age of 47 years. The most commonly reported symptoms included pain, sensory/neurological disturbances, psychological distress, and gastrointestinal symptoms (Table 1).

> **Practical pointer**
>
> Fibromyalgia patients characteristically report a wide variety of non-pain symptoms, including neurological disturbances, gastrointestinal, chronic fatigue, and psychological distress.

Table 1 Top 12 symptoms reported by people with fibromyalgia (Bennett [2])

Currently active symptoms	Percentage people with fibromyalgia reporting
Low-back pain	63
Recurrent headaches	47
Arthritis	46
Muscle spasm	46
Tingling	46
Balance disturbance	45
Irritable bowel syndrome	44
Numbness	44
Chronic fatigue	40
Bloating	40
Depression	40
Anxiety	38

A survey of 196 fibromyalgia patients showed that most fibromyalgia patients need more information to better understand fibromyalgia [3]. Fibromyalgia patients' attitudes about their condition, however, makes them excellent candidates for medical treatment, as most fibromyalgia patients are open to treatment, eager to comply with prescribed therapies, and hopeful for treatment benefit. Most patients with fibromyalgia believe:

- Fibromyalgia symptoms will likely be chronic
- Fibromyalgia symptoms are expected to fluctuate over time
- Fibromyalgia will have severe impact on physical, social, and psychological functioning

- There is a lot fibromyalgia patients can do personally to help control their symptoms
- Medical treatments are likely to be effective in decreasing their symptoms

Furthermore, patients did not endorse many negative emotions, such as anger, related to their fibromyalgia diagnosis. Healthcare providers, therefore, should be encouraged that, despite the wide assortment of complaints verbalized by fibromyalgia patients, these patients are generally engaged and expectant of good outcome with treatment.

Epidemiology of Fibromyalgia

Fibromyalgia affects about 2–3% of adults in the Americas and Europe [4–8]. Similar to other rheumatologic conditions, the prevalence is substantially lower in China at about 0.05% [9] (Fig. 1). Women are more likely to be affected with fibromyalgia. Interestingly, the prevalence of fibromyalgia remains relatively

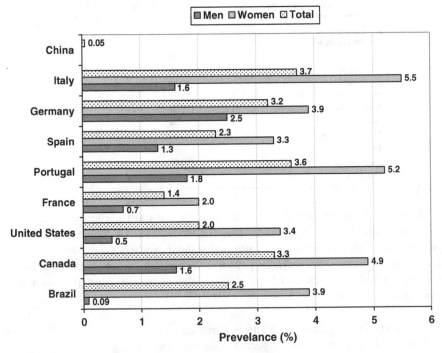

Fig. 1 Prevalence of fibromyalgia (based on Senna [4], McNally [7], Lawrence [6], Zeng [9], Branco [8]). Due to the low total prevalence in China (0.05%), gender differences were not available

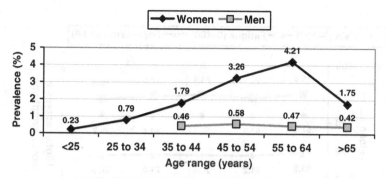

Fig. 2 Prevalence of fibromyalgia with age (based on McNally [7]). Sufficient data were not available to calculate prevalence in men before age 35

stable in men across their lifetimes, while the prevalence increases in women, peaking between ages 55–64 years old, and then declining in women ≥65 years old (Fig. 2) [7].

Practical pointer

Fibromyalgia affects about 2–3% of adults, with women affected about three times more often than men. Peak prevalence is between 55 and 64 years old.

Long-term prognosis of fibromyalgia was evaluated in a 5-year study in which female patients with fibromyalgia and no other chronic health conditions were interviewed annually [10]. Retention in the study was good with 287 women initially evaluated (average age = 47 years, average disease duration = 5 years). A total of 241 women completed at least two interviews and 211 completed all 5 years of assessment. Significant improvements were noted over time in fatigue, function, and depression score, although pain did not change significantly (Fig. 3).

Co-morbid Conditions

A diversity of other rheumatologic, medical, and psychological conditions is co-morbid with fibromyalgia. Using a large insurance claims database in the United States, the prevalence of concomitant illnesses was compared between patients with and without fibromyalgia [11]. Risk ratios >1 were used to identify co-morbid illness occurring with greater than expected prevalence among fibromyalgia patients (Fig. 4). Medical and psychological conditions were co-morbid in both genders with fibromyalgia. A detailed description of the most commonly occurring co-morbid conditions is provided in the chapters "Headache," "Chronic Fatigue Syndrome,"

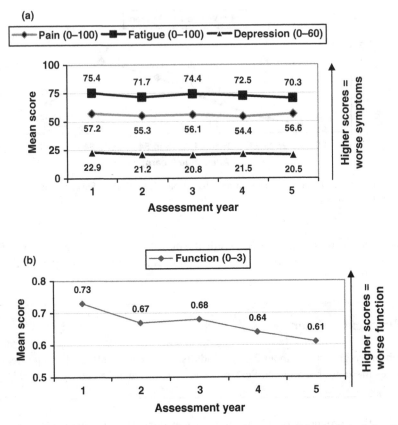

Fig. 3 Long-term outcome in fibromyalgia patients (based on Reisine [10]). (**a**) Pain, fatigue, and depression, (**b**) function

"Irritable Bowel Syndrome," "Sleep Disturbance," "Depression and Anxiety," and "Obesity and Metabolic Syndrome."

Autonomic dysfunction is also common among fibromyalgia patients. A syndrome that shares many features with fibromyalgia and may occur co-morbidly is postural orthostatic tachycardia syndrome (POTS). Normally, mild, asymptomatic cardiovascular changes occur when assuming an upright posture, with an immediate loss of about 500 mL of blood from the thorax to the abdomen and lower extremities and a 10–25% shift of plasma volume from vasculature to interstitial tissues. Venous return to the heart decreases and compensatory sympathetic activation occurs, causing a transient increase in heart rate during the first minute of about 10–20 beats per minute and systemic vasoconstriction with an approximate 5 mm Hg increase in diastolic blood pressure. POTS syndrome is defined as orthostatic tachycardia greater than expected from normal physiological changes that occurs without hypotension (Box 2). POTS exhibits circadian variability with the most extreme drop in heart rate occurring in the morning, so diagnostic testing should ideally be performed in the morning. Dark red mottling of the legs may

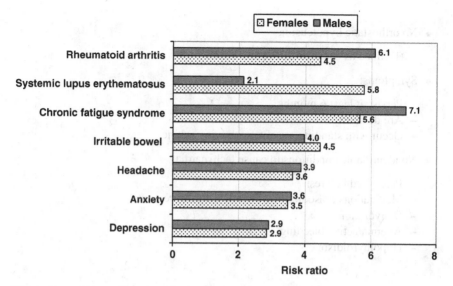

Fig. 4 Co-morbid conditions and fibromyalgia (based on Weir [11]). All of the conditions in the graph were co-morbid with fibromyalgia, except for systemic lupus erythematosus in men, which failed to achieve statistical significance due to wide data variability (95% confidence interval = 0.29–15.74)

be noted after standing for about 5 min. A variety of symptoms are commonly reported in patients with POTS (Box 3). The Mayo Clinic published data on a relatively large sample of POTS patients ($N = 152$), with the most commonly reported symptoms being light headedness or dizziness (78%), palpitations (75%), presyncope (61%), exercise intolerance (53%, heat intolerance (53%), weakness (50%), and fatigue (48%) [12]. POTS typically occurs between 12 and 51 years old, with women affected four to five times more often than men. POTS syndrome has been reported to occur in many patients with fibromyalgia, although good epidemiological data are lacking [13]. In an observational cohort study, POTS was identified in 9% of a control population vs. 27% with chronic fatigue syndrome [14]. Treatment is generally conservative and aerobic exercise should be encouraged as deconditioning at least worsens POTS and, in some cases, may have a causative influence (Box 4) [15].

Box 2 Criteria for POTS Diagnosis

- Orthostatic tachycardia

    - Heart rate increases ≥30 bpm OR to 120 bpm with standing 5–10 min
        - Only sinus tachycardia

- No orthostatic hypotension
  - (Defined as decrease 20/10 mm Hg BP)
- Symptoms:
  - Persist at least 6 months
  - Are disabling
  - Occur with standing, resolve with lying supine
- No identifiable conditions to cause tachycardia
  - Prolonged bed rest
  - Medications (vasodilators, diuretics, antidepressants)
  - Dehydration
  - Anemia/active bleeding
  - Hypothyroidism

Box 3 Common Symptoms with POTS

- Mental cloudiness
- Blurred/tunneled vision
- Shortness of breath
- Palpitations
- Tremulousness
- Chest pain
- Headache
- Lightheadedness
- Nausea
- Extreme fatigue
- Exercise intolerance

Box 4 POTS Treatment

- Hydration
  - 8–10 cups water daily
- Dietary salt
  - 200–300 mEq daily

- Waist-high elastic support hose
- Exercise
  - Aerobic and resistance training
    - 30 min, every other day

Orthostatic hypotension is also related to fibromyalgia. In an interesting study, 20 patients with fibromyalgia and 20 controls were subjected to tilt table testing [16]. An abnormal drop in blood pressure occurred in 60% of the fibromyalgia patients and none of the controls ($P<0.001$). Furthermore, all of the 18 fibromyalgia patients able to tolerate tilting for >10 min experienced aggravation of fibromyalgia pain during testing, while controls did not report pain.

Fibromyalgia Burden

Fibromyalgia can have substantial impact on patients' lives, despite the lack of limitations noted on physical examination in most fibromyalgia patients. A survey of women utilizing the National Fibromyalgia Association Web site ($N = 1,735$) reported substantial disability with fibromyalgia [17]. Most women reported difficulty with activities of daily living beyond personal care (Fig. 5).

Practical pointer

Fibromyalgia is associated with substantial disability. One in every 3–5 fibromyalgia patients reports a lot of difficulty with walking 1–2 blocks, climbing stairs, shopping, and carrying groceries.

Employment may also be negatively affected by fibromyalgia. One study compared work status in 136 fibromyalgia patients and age- and sex-matched controls who were being treating for non-rheumatologic conditions [18]. Work at the time of medical diagnosis was compared with current work situation at the time of study evaluation. Patients with fibromyalgia were significantly less likely to still be employed in the same job that they had at the time of their disease diagnosis compared with those without fibromyalgia (19% vs. 58%, $P<0.0001$). Job was lost due to the medical condition for 47% with fibromyalgia and 14% with other conditions. Furthermore, 7% of fibromyalgia and 5% of non-fibromyalgia patients additionally switched jobs due to their medical condition. In another

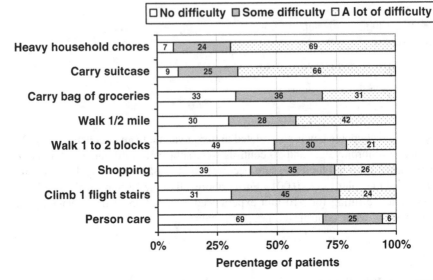

Fig. 5 Difficulty performing activities of daily living with fibromyalgia (based on Jones [17]). Heavy household chores would include scrubbing floors, vacuuming, or raking leaves

study, employees with fibromyalgia ($N = 8{,}513$) lost more work days annually compared with either employees with osteoarthritis ($N = 8{,}418$) or controls ($N = 7{,}260$) [19]. Both patient groups were actively involved with medical treatment for their respective conditions. Total days lost in 1 year were 30 days for employees with fibromyalgia vs. 26 for arthritis vs. 10 for controls (difference vs. fibromyalgia patients was significant for both arthritis and controls, $P<0.0001$). Consequently, fibromyalgia patients were absent from work on 15% of all possible work days over 1 year, about three times the loss seen with controls.

Despite the seemingly unremarkable physical examination findings in most patients with fibromyalgia, disease impact is similar for patients with fibromyalgia or those with rheumatoid arthritis, who likely have widespread pain but examinations with obvious physical findings. In an interesting study evaluating female outpatients with widespread pain from either fibromyalgia ($N = 62$) or rheumatoid arthritis ($N = 60$), sleep, physical function, and social function were similarly impaired in both groups [20]. Similarly, a comparison of the economic burden with two populations with chronic widespread pain (fibromyalgia [$N = 14{,}034$] and rheumatoid arthritis [$N = 7{,}965$]) showed substantial burden with both conditions [21]. Results of a 12-month analysis are shown in Fig. 6. In general, the burden of illness and direct costs with fibromyalgia were considerable and comparable to that seen with rheumatoid arthritis. Fibromyalgia patients utilized more healthcare visits, including emergency department, physician, and physical therapy visits, as well as inpatient hospitalizations and x-ray visits, compared with rheumatoid arthritis patients ($P<0.05$).

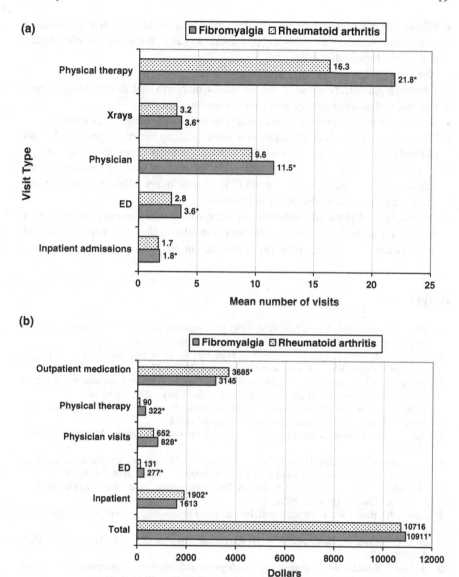

Fig. 6 Healthcare utilization and costs in patients with fibromyalgia vs. rheumatoid arthritis (based on Silverman [21]). (**a**) Healthcare appointments, (**b**) healthcare expenditures. *Significantly between-group differences, $P<0.05$

Summary

- Fibromyalgia is experienced as widespread pain, lasting ≥3 months, with at least 11 positive tender points on physical examination.

- Fibromyalgia patients characteristically report an abundance of non-pain-related symptoms, including neurological disturbances, gastrointestinal, chronic fatigue, and psychological distress.
- Non-pain symptoms tend to improve over time.
- Fibromyalgia affects about 2–3% of adults in North and South America and Europe, with a substantially lower prevalence in China.
- Women are about three times more likely to have fibromyalgia than men.
- Fibromyalgia prevalence increases in women, peaking between ages 54–64 years old and then decreasing. The prevalence in men is fairly constant across ages.
- Fibromyalgia is co-morbid with a diversity of medical and psychological conditions. Autonomic dysfunction (POTS) shares many clinical features with fibromyalgia and may also occur co-morbidly.
- Despite lack of physical limitations on examination noted in many patients with fibromyalgia, the burden of fibromyalgia is similar to that seen with rheumatoid arthritis, another chronic, widespread pain condition.

References

1. Wolfe F, Smythe HA, Yunus MB, et al. 1990 The American College of Rheumatology 1990 criteria for the classification of fibromyalgia. Arthritis Rheum. 1990;33:160–72.
2. Bennett RM, Jones J, Turk DC, Russell IJ, Matallana L. An internet survey of 2,596 people with fibromyalgia. BMC Musculoskeletal Disorders. 2007;8:27.
3. Van Ittersum MW, van Wilgen CP, Hilberdink WA, Groothoff JW, van der Schans CP. Illness perceptions in patients with fibromyalgia. Patient Educ Couns. 2009;74:53–60.
4. Senna ER, De Barros AL, Silva EO, et al. Prevalence of rheumatic diseases in Brazil: a study using the COPCORD approach. J Rheumatol. 2004;31:594–7.
5. Marcus DA. Fibromyalgia: diagnosis and treatment options. Gender Medicine. 2009;6: 139–51.
6. Lawrence RC, Fleson DT, Helmick CG, et al. Estimates of the prevalence of arthritis and other rheumatic conditions in the United States. Part II. Arthritis Rheum. 2008;58:26–35.
7. McNally JD, Matheson DA, Bakowsky VS. The epidemiology of self-reported fibromyalgia in Canada. Chronic Dis Can. 2006;27:9–16.
8. Branco JC, Bannwarth B, Failde I, et al. Prevalence of fibromyalgia: a survey of five European countries. Semin Arthritis Rheumat. 2010;39:448–53.
9. Zeng QY, Chen R, Darmawan J, et al. Rheumatic diseases in China. Arthritis Res Ther. 2008;10:R17.
10. Reisine S, Fifield J, Walsh, Forrest DD. Employment and health status changes among women with fibromyalgia: a five-year study. Arthritis Care Res. 2008;59:1735–41.
11. Weir PT, Harlan GA, Nkoy FL, et al. The incidence of fibromyalgia and its associated comorbidities: a population-based retrospective cohort study based on International Classification of Diseases, 9th Revision Codes. J Clin Rheumatol. 2006;12:124–8.
12. Thieben MJ, Sandroni P, Sletten DM, et al. Postural orthostatic tachycardia syndrome: the Mayo clinic experience. Mayo Clin Proc. 2007;82:308–13.
13. Staud R. Autonomic dysfunction in fibromyalgia syndrome: postural orthostatic tachycardia. Curr Rheumatol Rep. 2008;10:463–6.
14. Hoad A, Spickett G, Elliott J, Newton J. Postural orthostatic tachycardia syndrome is an underrecognized condition in chronic fatigue syndrome. QJM. 2008;101:961–5.
15. Joyner MJ, Masuki S. POTS versus deconditioning: the same or different? Clin Auton Res. 2008;18:300–7.

16. Bou-Holaigah I, Calkins H, Flynn JA, et al. Provocation of hypotension and pain during upright tilt table testing in adults with fibromyalgia. Clin Exp Rheumatol. 1997;15:239–46.
17. Jones J, Rutledge DN, Jones KD, Matallana L, Rooks DS. Self-assessed physical function levels of women with fibromyalgia: a national survey. Women's Health Issues. 2008;18: 406–12.
18. Al-Allaf. Work disability and health system utilization in patients with fibromyalgia syndrome. J Clin Rheumatol. 2007;13:199–201.
19. White LA, Birnbaum HG, Kaltenboeck A, et al. Employees with fibromyalgia: medical comorbidity, healthcare costs, and work loss. J Occup Environ Med. 2008;50:13–24.
20. Ofluoglu D, Berker N, Güven Z, et al. Quality of life in patients with fibromyalgia syndrome and rheumatoid arthritis. Clin Rheumatol 2005;24:490–2.
21. Silverman S, Dukes EM, Johnston SS, et al. The economic burden of fibromyalgia: comparative analysis with rheumatoid arthritis. Curr Med Res Opin. 2009;25:829–40.

Pathophysiology of Fibromyalgia

Key Chapter Points

- A variety of factors have been implicated in the pathophysiology of fibromyalgia, including changes in neural structure and function, muscular physiology, hormonal factors, inflammatory markers, and genetic influences.
- Fibromyalgia patients are more sensitive to painful stimulation, due to both peripheral and central sensitization.
- Increased sensitivity to pain is linked to reductions in brain activity in descending inhibitory pathways.
- Growth hormone deficiency and thyroid autoimmunity may be linked to fibromyalgia symptoms.
- Fibromyalgia aggregates in families, although no clear fibromyalgia gene(s) has been identified.
- Patients with fibromyalgia beginning after trauma have greater distress and disability.

Keywords Central sensitization · Genetics · Growth hormone · Interleukin · Thyroid antibodies · Trauma

---

Case: Sara is a 32-year-old mother of three who has been complaining of widespread pain, migraines, irritable bowel syndrome, fatigue, and vague numbness for the last 5 years. "I was finally diagnosed with fibromyalgia 2 years ago, but I don't think my doctor really believes in fibromyalgia. He seems to think that my symptoms are just from me being anxious or depressed. I've already seen four doctors and each one just referred me to a psychiatrist when he heard I have fibromyalgia. I'm beginning to wonder if fibromyalgia is something real or just in my head. I wish someone could figure out what's causing fibromyalgia!"

Implementation of standardized and widely accepted classification criteria of fibromyalgia by the American College of Rheumatology in 1990 has allowed

D.A. Marcus, A. Deodhar, *Fibromyalgia*, DOI 10.1007/978-1-4419-1609-9_3,
© Springer Science+Business Media, LLC 2011

research into the pathophysiology of fibromyalgia. While early descriptions of fibromyalgia symptoms focused on psychological factors, current research into the pathophysiology of fibromyalgia has identified a plethora of biological dysfunction supporting categorizing fibromyalgia as the consequence of primarily physical rather than purely emotional dysfunction. As with many types of chronic, nonmalignant pain, current research suggests an important role for aberrant pain processing with peripheral and central sensitization in fibromyalgia patients. Abnormalities of a diversity of factors likely influence the development of fibromyalgia symptoms, including neural structure and function, muscular physiology, hormonal factors, inflammatory markers, and genetic influences. The role of trauma in fibromyalgia pathogenesis remains controversial. Researchers have recently begun to identify factors that may help identify those individuals who may be more susceptible to physiological changes that result in the development of fibromyalgia.

Nerve Abnormalities

Evaluations of structural abnormalities have shown both peripheral neural changes in the skin and central changes in the brain. While structural changes imply neural dysfunction, functional studies are needed to understand the possible clinical significance of neural changes. Functional studies have consistently demonstrated enhanced neural sensitivity to painful and non-painful stimuli or central sensitization that is likely a key factor in the development of fibromyalgia pain and excessive sensitivity to most sensory stimuli. Studies show that peripheral injury can result in pain hypersensitivity and central sensitization through activation of both neurons and glia [1]. These changes are likely important for the development of persistent pain complaints in the absence of ongoing injury for a variety of chronic pain conditions, including fibromyalgia.

Structural Changes

Data evaluating structural changes of neural tissue are limited; however, available research does suggest morphological changes that might be linked to neural sensitization. Due to increased peripheral sensitivity noticed in fibromyalgia patients, studies have evaluated changes in neural structures in the skin. One research group evaluated skin biopsies from 13 fibromyalgia patients and 5 controls; Schwann cell ballooning, axon peripheralization, smaller axon size, and simplified folding structures were identified in unmyelinated neurons of fibromyalgia patients when evaluated using electron microscopy [2]. Additional work by this same group linked these morphological changes to peripheral sensitization of N-methyl-D-aspartate

(NMDA) receptors. NMDA receptors play a critical role in temporal summation or "wind-up," a key mechanism in the development of chronic pain. NMDA receptors are present in both the dorsal root ganglion and the skin; glutamate, an important excitatory neurotransmitter and pain modulator, binds to NMDA NR2 subunits. Skin NMDA receptor subtypes were evaluated in the skin of 11 female fibromyalgia patients and 8 healthy matched controls [3]. NR2D receptors were increased in fibromyalgia patients (159 vs.100, $P = 0.016$), with receptor expression correlated to disease duration ($P = 0.046$). Peripheral neural changes are additionally supported by data showing upregulation of both delta- and kappa-opioid receptors, with concentrations significantly higher in fibromyalgia patients than in controls ($P<0.01$) [4]. Interestingly, opioid receptor mRNA in muscle is similar for fibromyalgia patients and controls.

Practical pointer

Peripheral sensitization is suggested in the skin of fibromyalgia patients with increased NMDA receptors and upregulation of opioid receptors.

Subtle changes in the brain have also been identified by comparing brain volumes in patients with fibromyalgia and controls [5]. In one study, total brain volume and total gray and white matter volumes were similar between groups; however, fibromyalgia patients demonstrated significantly reduced gray matter in the inferior frontal gyrus ($P = 0.04$), amygdala ($P = 0.004$), and anterior cingulated cortex ($P = 0.004$). These areas are known to be important for pain processing [6]. Although the functional significance of these findings was not tested in this study, the authors postulated that volume reductions may predispose patients to the development of central sensitization believed to be important in pain perception and expression in fibromyalgia (see below). A similar study likewise showed reductions in gray matter volume in these same regions in fibromyalgia patients and correlated these reductions with dopamine metabolism, suggesting a possible important functional impact from these gray matter volume changes [7].

Practical pointer

Subtle changes in gray matter in the brain affect areas important for pain processing.

Functional Changes

Anecdotally, fibromyalgia patients often endorse having an increased sensitivity to stimulation being perceived as painful and a seemingly exaggerated perception of discomfort to stimuli that would not produce pain in normal controls. Physiological studies confirm this subjective report of increased pain sensitivity with fibromyalgia. Experimental studies show that the temperatures required to perceive a stimulus as either cold or hot are nearly identical for fibromyalgia patients and controls; however, temperature changes required to produce a pain perception are substantially lower for both cold pain ($P<0.001$) and heat pain ($P<0.01$) in fibromyalgia patients (Fig. 1) [8]. Repeated stimulus exposure results in increased pain sensations, or wind-up, in fibromyalgia patients, an example of central sensitization. Fibromyalgia patients and healthy controls both report higher pain ratings after repeated exposures to heat; however, the degree of wind-up, temporal summation, and prolonged after sensations (suggestive of increased central sensitivity to pain messages) is significantly greater in fibromyalgia subjects [9].

Practical pointer

Fibromyalgia patients are more sensitive to painful stimuli due to central sensitization.

Both subjective and objective pain responses differ in fibromyalgia patients compared with controls. When exposed to the same painful stimulus, fibromyalgia patients report greater subjective pain perception. Objective functional magnetic resonance imaging (fMRI) has confirmed that this increased subjective sensitivity is accompanied by decreased brain activity in areas serving descending pain

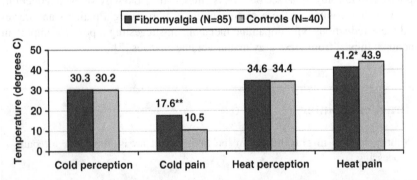

Fig. 1 Enhanced perception of cold and hot pain in fibromyalgia (based on Desmeules [8]). Between-group differences were significant for pain: $*P < 0.01$; $**P < 0.001$

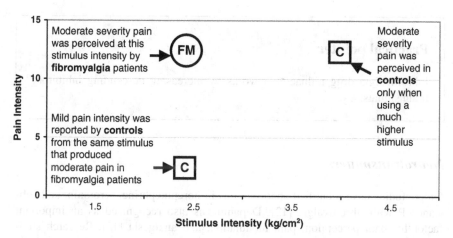

Fig. 2 Pain threshold comparison between fibromyalgia patients and controls (based on Gracely [10]). Pain scale was from 0 (no pain) to 15 (maximum severity pain). Moderate pain was represented by a score of 11. C=average control response; FM=average fibromyalgia patient response

inhibitory pathways. In a frequently quoted study, Gracely and colleagues measured the severity of a pain stimulus required to result in a moderate severity pain response in fibromyalgia patients and controls [10]. In order to produce a moderate level of pain perception, a 73% stronger stimulus was required for controls compared with fibromyalgia patients (Fig. 2). The physiological importance of this difference was demonstrated in fMRI studies used to calculate difference in brain activation between touch and pain stimulation. Brain activation was comparable when using that level of stimulation required to produce a subjective report of moderate severity pain in both fibromyalgia patients and controls. Utilizing the same stimulation intensity, however, resulted in significantly greater activation in fibromyalgia patients compared with controls ($P<0.05$). This important study shows that there is a physiological basis for the reports of increased pain perception to lower levels of pain stimulus intensity in fibromyalgia patients. Furthermore, fibromyalgia patients treated with milnacipran experience reduced pain and a parallel increase in brain activity in descending inhibitory pathways, confirming that milnacipran's effect occurs due to more than simply reduction in depressive symptoms [11].

Practical pointer

The validity of fibromyalgia patients' reports of increased sensitivity to pain is supported by functional MRI studies showing enhanced brain activation or central sensitization.

Practical pointer

Fibromyalgia drug milnacipran works by increasing descending inhibitory brain signals.

Neurotransmitters

Older studies have identified abnormalities in norepinephrine, serotonin, and substance P with fibromyalgia [12]. Dopamine is also recognized as an important factor for pain perception, pain modulation, and analgesia [13]. Research studies have identified both dopamine abnormalities in fibromyalgia and symptomatic improvement after treatment with dopaminergic drugs [14]. For example, in a double-blind, placebo-controlled study ($N = 60$), dopamine agonist pramipexole significantly improved pain in fibromyalgia patients [15]. Pain severity was reduced by at least 50% in 42% treated with 4.5 mg pramipexole daily vs. 14% with placebo. Improvements in function and fatigue likewise favored pramipexole ($P<0.03$).

Musculoskeletal Abnormalities

Muscle Dysfunction

Muscles can be divided into slow contraction, red Type I fibers important for static muscle tone and posture and the fast contraction white Type II fibers that produce high power for short duration. While fibromyalgia is not considered primarily a disorder of muscles (like myofascial pain), dysfunction of muscle histology, metabolism, and function (Box 1) may have important roles in both pain and fatigue in fibromyalgia patients [16].

Box 1 Muscle Abnormalities in Fibromyalgia Patients (Based on Park [16])

- Microscopic changes
    - Ragged red fibers
    - Abnormal mitochondria
    - Abnormal cell membranes
    - Type II fiber atrophy

- Abnormalities in muscle metabolism
  - 15% decreased ATP and phosphocreatinine
- 25–60% reduced contraction strength
- Reduced aerobic endurance

Muscular abnormalities were evaluated in a recent study testing 100 fibromyalgia patients and 50 controls with surface electromyography of the vastus medialis muscle [17]. Absolute values of median spectral frequency (a fatigue index) and conduction velocity were lower at baseline and after muscle contraction in fibromyalgia patients. Interestingly, however, the percentage reduction after contraction was less in the fibromyalgia patients. These changes led researchers to speculate that a reduction in the proportion of Type II muscle fibers or possibly abnormal fiber recruitment in fibromyalgia patients led to this difference in response to muscle activation.

Practical pointer

Deficits in Type II muscle fibers may contribute to weakness and fatigue in fibromyalgia.

Co-contraction of antagonist muscles can result in increased muscle tension and pain in chronic widespread pain [18]. In an interesting study, researchers identified excessive recruitment of antagonist muscles when fibromyalgia patients attempted to utilize voluntary muscles compared with non-pain controls [19]. After fatiguing the muscle, co-contraction in the upper arm was significantly more pronounced in fibromyalgia patients compared with controls ($P = 0.01$). In the Fig. 3, ratios of

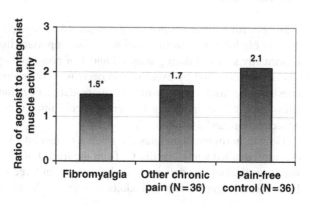

Fig. 3 Co-contraction in upper arm (based on Jegede [19]). Smaller ratios signify greater degrees of co-contraction. Difference between fibromyalgia patients and controls was significant ($P = 0.01$)

activity of agonist to antagonist muscle are shown. When abnormal co-contraction of antagonist muscles was higher, the ratio was lower. So a lower number signifies more co-contraction. There was numerically more co-contraction with fibromyalgia patients than patients with other chronically painful conditions, although this difference was not significant.

Cervical Spine Abnormalities

Transient cervical nerve root compression in rats has been shown to result in persistent, bilateral allodynia, possibly serving as a model for fibromyalgia [20]. Co-morbid cervical spinal cord compression has also been reported in fibromyalgia patients. In a retrospective chart review of 107 patients referred to rheumatology, 53 were diagnosed with fibromyalgia, 22 with non-fibromyalgia chronic widespread pain, and 32 with inflammatory connective tissue disease [21]. Flexion-extension MRI was obtained in 70 patients, with Chiari I malformation identified in two fibromyalgia patients and cervical cord abutment or compression (generally with extension) in 52 patients (35 of 49 imaged fibromyalgia patients [71%] and 17 of 20 imaged non-fibromyalgia chronic widespread pain patients [85%].) These data support findings from an earlier study of 270 fibromyalgia patients examined for cervical myelopathy [22]. In this study, both symptomatic reports and neurological findings worsened in 88% of patients during neck extension. In addition, the C5/6 spinal canal diameter was identified as stenotic ($\leq$10 mm) during extension in 46% of patients. The significance of these findings remains controversial; however, in one study, fibromyalgia patients with clinically diagnosed cervical myelopathy experienced improvement in fibromyalgia symptoms following treatment of their myelopathy [23].

Hormonal Factors

Growth Hormone

While growth hormone is primarily considered to be important for the development process of children, growth hormone is also important in adults. Growth hormone is primarily secreted during stages 3 and 4 of non-rapid eye movement sleep, with levels also increased by exercise and decreased by chronic stress, depression, and obesity [24]. Adults with growth hormone deficiency share many clinical features with fibromyalgia, including low energy, cold intolerance, impaired memory and concentration, and dysthmia [24].

Growth hormone stimulates the release of insulin-like growth factor-1 (IGF-1, previously called somatomedin C) from the liver. IGF-1 is deficient in most adults with growth hormone deficiency and about one in three fibromyalgia patients [25]. Both fibromyalgia patients and adults with growth hormone deficiency share a poor growth hormone response to non-insulin stimulation testing (e.g., acute exercise), while response to insulin tolerance testing or arginine/growth hormone releasing hormone stimulation is impaired with adult growth hormone deficiency but normal with fibromyalgia [24]. This would indicate that the growth hormone deficiency in fibromyalgia is probably linked to hypothalamic rather than pituitary dysfunction. There is indirect evidence of increased hypothalamic somatostatin tone in patients with FM, which, in turn, reduces the release of growth hormone by the pituitary [26].

Practical pointer

Fibromyalgia shares features of growth hormone deficiency, including reduced IGF-1 and clinical symptoms of low energy, cold intolerance, impaired memory and concentration, and dysthmia.

Some drugs used to treat fibromyalgia, like tricyclic antidepressants and opioids, stimulate growth hormone, while selective serotonin reuptake inhibitors decrease growth hormone and IGF-1. Treatment trials specifically designed to treat growth hormone deficiency in fibromyalgia have produced mixed results. An early study in which women with fibromyalgia and low IGF-1 levels ($N = 50$) were randomized to daily subcutaneous injections of growth hormone or placebo for 9 months showed increases in IGF-1 levels and significantly reduced fibromyalgia symptoms ($P<0.04$) and tender point score ($P<0.03$) with growth hormone therapy after about 6 months of treatment [27]. Symptoms worsened after discontinuing growth hormone injections. Conversely, efforts to improve growth hormone via exercise in fibromyalgia have not yielded positive results. A small 5-month study ($N = 26$) showed improved strength with exercise training in fibromyalgia patients, with no significant increase in either growth hormone or IGF-1 [28]. Likewise, a 6-month study ($N = 154$) evaluating exercise with or without pyridostigmine (shown to normalize acute growth hormone response to exercise) failed to show increases in IGF-1 [29]. Pain severity decreased by about 9% with placebo vs. 20% with exercise alone and 26% with exercise plus pyridostigmine [30]. This difference, however, did not achieve statistical significance.

Thyroid Function

Autoimmune thyroid disease occurs more commonly in patients with rheumatic disease [31]. In a survey of 65 patients with either hypo- or hyperthyroidism, one in three had fibromyalgia [31]. A study assessing thyroid function in 120 fibromyalgia patients found normal basal thyroid hormone, although thyroid antibodies were identified in 41% of patients vs. 15% of controls [32]. Those fibromyalgia patients with thyroid autoimmunity showed a higher percentage of dry eyes (56% with anti-bodies vs. 37% without antibodies, $P<0.05$), burning or pain with urination (36% vs. 10%, $P<0.01$), allodynia (the perception of normally non-painful touch stimuli as painful; 74% vs. 32%, $P<0.01$), blurred vision (49% vs. 23%, $P<0.01$), and sore throat (44% vs. 17%, $P<0.01$). This study confirmed a report from an earlier study identifying significantly more prevalent thyroid autoimmunity in euthyroid patients with fibromyalgia (34%) or rheumatoid arthritis (30%) compared with healthy controls (19%, $P<0.05$) [33]. That study correlated thyroid autoimmunity with fibromyalgia duration (8.3 years if thyroid antibodies were present vs. 4.5 years if antibody negative, $P = 0.013$), previous psychiatric disease (50% vs. 30%, $P = 0.024$), co-morbid headache (27% vs. 12%, $P = 0.029$), and dry mouth (41% vs. 20%, $P = 0.013$).

Practical pointer

Fibromyalgia is linked to an increased prevalence of thyroid autoimmunity. Patients with thyroid antibodies have increased reports of dry eyes, allodynia, and headache.

Neuroendocrine Abnormalities

Altered activity of the hypothalamic–pituitary–adrenal axis may also contribute to fibromyalgia symptomatology. A recent review showed that, while adrenal gland size is normal in fibromyalgia patients, a variety of neuroendocrine abnormalities have been identified [34]:

- Decreased response of ACTH and epinephrine to hypoglycemia
- Decreased peak cortical response to ACTH
- Decreased 11-deoxycortisol after metyrapone test.

The hypothalamic–pituitary–adrenal axis may be less resilient than normal in fibromyalgia patients, which may contribute to the impaired response to stress that many of these patients exhibit and the role that stress can play in aggravating fibromyalgia symptoms [35, 36].

Inflammatory Markers

Proinflammatory cytokines have been shown to affect neural excitability and facilitate pain transmission [37]. An inflammatory response has been shown to activate NMDA receptors and microglia proliferation, which may explain the development of hypersensitivity and chronic pain complaints [38]. Cytokines, like interleukins

(IL), have also been postulated to play a role in fibromyalgia, although consistent changes have not been identified. Increased levels of IL-1, IL-2, IL-6, and IL-8 have been reported [39]. In a recent study, long-term changes in IL-8 were monitored in fibromyalgia patients [40]. At baseline, IL-8 levels were significantly higher among fibromyalgia patients compared with controls (11.05 vs. 4.96 pg/mL, $P<0.001$). Over the course of multidisciplinary treatment, IL-8 levels declined to normal levels, with decreasing IL-8 correlating with reduced pain severity.

Genetics

A number of studies have suggested a strong familial aggregation of fibromyalgia, with some studies suggesting an autosomal dominant inheritance pattern [41]. More recently, Arnold and colleagues analyzed familial aggregation in 78 fibromyalgia patients and their 533 relatives and 40 rheumatoid arthritis patients and their 272 relatives [42]. The odds of having fibromyalgia were 8.5 times higher among people with a relative with fibromyalgia compared with those having a relative with rheumatoid arthritis. Furthermore, relatives of fibromyalgia patients displayed significantly higher tender point counts compared with relatives of rheumatoid arthritis patients, although the sum of pain readings from all points tested (tender point scores) was significantly lower among relatives of fibromyalgia patients ($P<0.0001$). Data for those relatives available for interview and assessment ($N = 146$ for fibromyalgia patients and $N = 72$ for rheumatoid arthritis patients) are shown in Fig. 4.

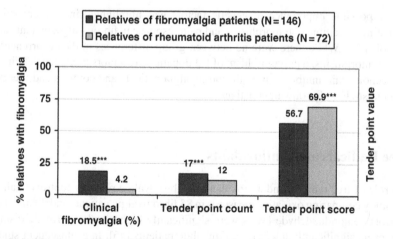

Fig. 4 Aggregation of fibromyalgia diagnosis and tender points in relatives of patients with fibromyalgia vs. rheumatoid arthritis (based on Arnold [42]). The mean tender point count is the average number of positive tender points. The mean tender point score is the average sum total of severity scores obtained at all 18 tender points tested using dolorimetry testing and 4 kg pressure. Differences between groups were significant ***$P<0.001$

Researchers in Sweden evaluated pain data collected on 15,950 twin pairs $\geq$42 years old in the Swedish Twin Registry [43]. In this study, chronic widespread pain was diagnosed using the American College of Rheumatology criteria for fibromyalgia, although no physical examinations were performed. Among women, concordance rate was 0.29 among monozygotic twin pairs and 0.16 among dizygotic twins. Among men, concordance rate was 0.14 among monozygotic twins and 0.05 among dizygotic twins. Overall, genetic and shared environment each explained about half of the variation in the occurrence of chronic widespread pain in this study, suggesting a modest genetic influence.

Practical pointer

Fibromyalgia tends to run in families, although genetics probably accounts for only half of the variation in occurrence of fibromyalgia.

A variety of possible candidate genes has been linked to fibromyalgia [44]:

- HLA DR4 antigen
- Serotonin transporter
- Cathechol-*O*-methyl transferase
- Dopamine receptors
- Substance P receptor NK1

The possible importance of genetic factors was highlighted in a recent study evaluating dopamine polymorphisms and pain response in fibromyalgia patients and controls [45]. While there were no between-group differences in the occurrence of D3 polymorphisms, a polymorphism of D3 dopamine receptors predicted deficits in endogenous pain inhibition in both fibromyalgia patients and controls and thermal pain threshold in fibromyalgia patients.

Free Radicals and Antioxidants

The role of free radicals and antioxidants in fibromyalgia remains controversial. In one study comparing oxidative measures in 85 fibromyalgia patients and 80 matched controls, malondialdehyde levels were significantly higher and superoxide dismutase levels significantly lower in fibromyalgic patients [46]. In a subsequent study, total antioxidant capacity was significantly lower in 20 fibromyalgia patients vs. 20 controls (1.5 vs. 1.9 mm Trolox equiv/L, $P = 0.001$), while total peroxide level was higher in fibromyalgia patients (37.4 vs. 33.0 micromol H_2O_2/L, $P = 0.01$) [47].

Furthermore, pain was negatively correlated with antioxidant capacity, supporting a possible contributory role in fibromyalgia symptoms.

Trauma

The role of physical trauma and fibromyalgia remains highly controversial [48]. A case-controlled study evaluated the occurrence of trauma in the 6 months prior to developing fibromyalgia symptoms [49]. Trauma was reported in 39% of the fibromyalgia patients vs. 24% of controls ($P = 0.007$). Among individual types of injury, surgery ($P = 0.004$) and work injury ($P = 0.015$) were significantly more likely to occur prior to the onset of fibromyalgia. In one study, fibromyalgia beginning after trauma was linked to increased healthcare seeking and disability, but not pain severity [50]. Another study controlling for possible financial compensation (including disability and litigation) reported that fibromyalgia beginning after trauma was associated with greater pain severity, disability, and psychological distress [51]. These studies suggest that those patients reporting fibromyalgia beginning after trauma may require more aggressive treatment to minimize disability.

Practical pointer

Fibromyalgia beginning after trauma is linked to greater distress, disability, and utilization of healthcare. Therefore, post-trauma fibromyalgia may require more aggressive treatment.

Predictive Factors

A comparison of 287 women with fibromyalgia treated in a rheumatology clinic and 287 non-fibromyalgia controls who were patients in an ears nose and throat clinic of the same hospital identified predictive factors for fibromyalgia [52]. Several demographic factors, the occurrence of psychological distress, and more frequent abuse as an adult by a non-partner were each significantly linked to increased risk for having the diagnosis of fibromyalgia (Fig. 5). Interestingly, neither abuse as an adult by an intimate partner nor childhood abuse was linked to increased fibromyalgia risk. Therefore, fibromyalgia patients should be routinely screened for the presence of depression and anxiety and the occurrence of abuse.

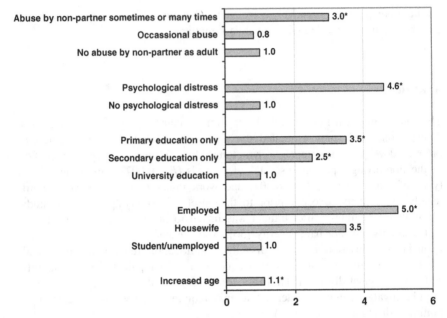

Fig. 5 Independent risk factors for fibromyalgia (based on Ruiz-Pérez [52]). Independent risk factors with 95% CI not including 1.0 are shown with asterisks

Summary

- Fibromyalgia patients are more sensitive to painful stimulation, due to both peripheral and central sensitization. Pain perception is higher and functional magnetic resonance imaging shows that this increased subjective sensitivity is accompanied by a decreased activity in brain descending pain inhibitory pathways.
- Changes in neurotransmitters, including dopamine, suggest possible treatment options.
- Muscle abnormalities include reductions in Type II fibers, abnormal muscle metabolism, and excessive agonist–antagonist co-contraction. These changes may result in weakness, fatigue, and muscle pain in fibromyalgia patients.
- Inflammatory cytokines are elevated in patients with fibromyalgia, with levels decreasing with fibromyalgia treatment in conjunction with improvements in pain severity.
- Growth hormone deficiency related to hypothalamic dysfunction has been postulated to play a role in fibromyalgia, although treatment studies have yielded mixed results.
- Thyroid autoimmunity is more prevalent in fibromyalgia and is associated with an increase in a variety of symptoms, including dry eyes, allodynia, and headache.

- Because psychological distress and abuse occur more commonly in fibromyalgia patients, all patients reporting chronic widespread pain should be screened for depression, anxiety, and abuse.

References

1. Ren K, Dubner R. Neuron-glia crosstalk gets serious: role in pain hypersensitivity. Curr Opin Ananes. 2008;21:570–9.
2. Kim SH, Kim DH, Oh DH, Clauw DJ. Characteristic electron microscopic findings in the skin of patients with fibromyalgia: preliminary study. Clin Rheumatol. 2008;27:219–23.
3. Kim SH, Jang TJ, Moon IS. Increased expression of N-methyl-D-aspartate receptor subunit 2D in the skin of patients with fibromyalgia. J Rheumatol. 2006;33:785–8.
4. Salemi S, Aeschlimann A, Wollina U, et al. Up-regulation of delta-opioid receptors and kappa-opioid receptors in the skin of fibromyalgia patients. Arthritis Rheum. 2007;56:2464–6.
5. Burgmer M, Gaubitz M, Konrad C, et al. Decreased gray matter volumes in the cingulo-frontal cortex and the amygdala in patients with fibromyalgia. Psychosom Med. 2009;71:566–73.
6. Moisset X, Bouhassira D, Denis D, et al. Anatomical connections between brain areas activated during rectal distension in healthy volunteers: A visceral pain network. Eur J Pain. 2010;14:142–8.
7. Wood PB, Glabus MF, Simpson R, Patterson JC. Changes in gray matter density in fibromyalgia: correlation with dopamine metabolism. J Pain. 2009;10:609–18.
8. Desmeules JA, Cedraschi C, Rapiti E, et al. Neurophysiologic evidence for a central sensitization in patients with fibromyalgia. Arthritis Rheum. 2003;48:1420–9.
9. Staud R, Vierck CJ, Cannon RL, Mauderli AP, Price DD. Abnormal sensitization and temporal summation of second pain (wind-up) in patients with fibromyalgia syndrome. Pain. 2001;91:165–75.
10. Gracely RH, Petzke F, Wolf JM, Clauw DJ. Functional magnetic resonance imaging evidence of augmented pain processing in fibromyalgia. Arthritis Rheum. 2002;46:1333–43.
11. Mainguy Y. Functional magnetic resonance imagery (fMRI) in fibromyalgia and the response to milnacipran. Hum Psychopharmacol. 2009;24:S19–23.
12. Bernstein C, Marcus DA. Fibromyalgia: current concepts in diagnosis, pathogenesis, and treatment. Pain Med News. 2008;6:8–19.
13. Wood PB. Role of central dopamine in pain and analgesia. Expert Rev Neurother. 2008;8: 781–97.
14. Wood PB, Holman AJ. An elephant among us: the role of dopamine in the pathophysiology of fibromyalgia. J Rheumatol. 2009;36:221–4.
15. Holman AJ, Myers RR.A randomized, double-blind, placebo-controlled trial of pramipexole, a dopamine agonist, in patients with fibromyalgia receiving concomitant medications. Arthritis Rheum. 2005;52:2495–505.
16. Park JH, Niermann KJ, Olsen NJ. Evidence for metabolic abnormalities in the muscles of patients with fibromyalgia. Curr Rheumatol Rep. 2000;2:131–40.
17. Bazzichi L, Dini M, Rossi A, et al. Muscle modifications in fibromyalgia patients revealed by surface electromyography (SEMG) analysis. BMC Musculoskelet Disord. 2009;10:36.
18. Thompson J. Myofascial pain syndrome and fibromyalgia: a critical assessment and alternative view. Clin J Pain. 1998;14:82–4.
19. Jegede AB, Gilbert C, Tulkin SR. Muscle characteristics of persons with fibromyalgia syndrome. Neurorehabilitation. 2008;23:217–30.
20. Hubbard RD, Winkelstein BA. Transient cervical nerve root compression in the rat induces bilateral forepaw allodynia and spinal glial activation: mechanical factors in painful neck injuries. Spine. 2005;30:1924–32.

21. Holman AJ. Positional cervical spinal cord compression and fibromyalgia: a novel comorbidity with important diagnostic and treatment implications. J Pain. 2008;9:613–22.

22. Heffez DS, Ross RE, Shade-Zeldow Y et al. Clinical evidence for cervical myelopathy due to Chiari malformation and spinal stenosis in a non-randomized group of patients with the diagnosis of fibromyalgia. Eur Spine J. 2004;13:516–23.

23. Heffez DS, Ross RE, Shade-Zeldow Y, et al. Treatment of cervical myelopathy in patients with the fibromyalgia syndrome: outcomes and implications. Eur Spine J. 2007;16:1423–33.

24. Jones KD, Deodhar P, Lorentzen A, Bennett RM, Deodhar AA. Growth hormone perturbations in fibromyalgia: a review. Semin Arthritis Rheum. 2007;36:357–79.

25. Bennett RM, Cook DM, Clark SR, Burckhardt CS, Campbell SM. Hypothalamic-pituitary-insulin-like growth factor-1 axis dysfunction in patients with fibromyalgia. J Rheumatol. 1997;24:1384–9.

26. Paiva ES, Deodhar AA, Jones K, Bennett R. Impaired growth hormone secretion in fibromyalgia patients: Evidence for augmented hypothalamic somatostatin tone. Arthritis Rheum. 2002;46:1344–50.

27. Bennett RM, Clark SC, Walczyk J. A randomized, double-blind, placebo-controlled study of growth hormone in the treatment of fibromyalgia. Am J Med. 1998;104:227–31.

28. Valkeinen H, Häkkinen K, Pakarinen A, et al. Muscle hypertrophy, strength development, and serum hormones during strength training in elderly women with fibromyalgia. Scand J Rheumatol. 2005;34:309–14.

29. Jones KD, Deodhar AA, Burckhardt CS, et al. A combination of 6 months of treatment with pyridostigmine and triweekly exercise fails to improve insulin-like growth factor-I levels in fibromyalgia, despite improvement in the acute growth hormone response to exercise. J Rheumatol. 2007;34:1103–11.

30. Jones KD, Burckhardt CS, Deodhar AA, et al. A six-month randomized controlled trial of exercise and pyridostigmine in the treatment of fibromyalgia. Arthritis Rheum. 2008;58: 612–22.

31. Soy M, Guldiken S, Arikan E, Altun BU, Tuqrul A. Frequency of rheumatic diseases in patients with autoimmune thyroid disease. Rheumatol Int. 2007;27:575–7.

32. Bazzichi L, Rossi A, Giuliano T, et al. Association between thyroid autoimmunity and fibromyalgic disease severity. Clin Rheumatol. 2007;26:2115–20.

33. Pamuk ON, Cakir N. The frequency of thyroid antibodies in fibromyalgia patients and their relationship with symptoms. Clin Rheumatol. 2007;26:55–9.

34. Tanriverdi F, Karaca Z, Unluhizarci K, Kelestimur F. The hypothalamo-pituitary-adrenal axis in chronic fatigue syndrome and fibromyalgia syndrome. Stress. 2007;10:13–25.

35. Crofford LJ, Young EA, Engleberg NC, et al. Basal circadian and pulsatile ACTH and cortisol secretion in patients with fibromyalgia and/or chronic fatigue syndrome. Brain Behav Immun. 2004;18:314–25.

36. Crofford LJ. The hypothalamic-pituitary-adrenal stress axis in fibromyalgia and chronic fatigue syndrome. Z Rheumatol. 1998;57:67–71.

37. Schäfers M, Sorkin L. Effect of cytokines on neuronal excitability. Neurosci Lett. 2008;437:188–93.

38. Nair A, Bonneau RH. Stress-induced elevation of glucocorticoids increases microglia proliferation through NMDA receptor activation. J Neuroimmunology. 2006;171:72–85.

39. Thompson ME, Barkhuizen A. Fibromyalgia, hepatitis C infection, and the cytokine connection. Curr Pain Headache Rep. 2003;7:342–7.

40. Wang H, Buchner M, Moser MT, Daniel V, Schiltenwolf M. The role of IL-8 in patients with fibromyalgia: a prospective longitudinal study of 6 months. Clin J Pain. 2009;25:1–4.

41. Buskila D. Genetics of chronic pain states. Best Pract Res Clin Rheumatol. 2007;21: 535–47.

42. Arnold LM, Hudson JI, Hess EV et al. Family study of fibromyalgia. Arthritis Rheum. 2004;50:944–52.

43. Kato K, Sullivan PF, Evengård B, Pederson NL. Importance of genetic influences on chronic widespread pain. Arthritis Rheum. 2006;54:1682–6.
44. Ablin JN, Cohen H, Buskila D. Mechanisms of disease: genetics of fibromyalgia. Nat Clin Pract Rheumatol. 2006;2:671–8.
45. Potvin S, Larouche A, Normand E, et al. DRD3 Ser9Gly polymorphism is related to thermal pain perception and modulation in chronic widespread pain patients and healthy controls. J Pain. 2009;10:969–75.
46. Bagis S, Tamer L, Sahin G, et al. Free radicals and antioxidants in primary fibromyalgia: an oxidative stress disorder? Rheumatol Int. 2005;25:188–90.
47. Altindag O, Celik H. Total antioxidant capacity and the severity of the pain in patients with fibromyalgia. Redox Rep. 2006;11:131–5.
48. Sukenik S, Abu-Shakra M, Flusser D. Physical trauma and fibromyalgia – is there a true association? Harefuah. 2008;147:712–6.
49. Al-Allaf AW, Dunbar KL, Hallum NS, et al. A case-control study examining the role of physical trauma in the onset of fibromyalgia syndrome. Rheumatology. 2002;41:450–3.
50. Aaron LA, Bradley LA, Alarcón GS, et al. Perceived physical and emotional trauma as precipitating events in fibromyalgia. Associations with health care seeking and disability status but not pain severity. Arthritis Rheum. 1997;40:453–60.
51. Turk DC, Okifuji A, Starz TW, Sinclair JD. Effects of type of symptom onset on psychological distress in fibromyalgia syndrome patients. Pain. 1996;68:423–30.
52. Ruiz-Pérez I, Plazaola-Castaño J, Cáliz-Cáliz R, et al. Risk factors for fibromyalgia: the role of violence against women. Clin Rheumatol. 2009;28:777–86.

Assessment and Diagnosis

Key Chapter Points

- A tender point examine can be readily performed at the bedside using no special equipment.
- The presence and severity of common fibromyalgia symptoms should be assessed at the time of diagnosis and monitored during treatment.
- Screening for psychological distress should be performed in all fibromyalgia patients, including those not reporting depression or anxiety.
- The FibroFatigue Scale is an easy-to-administer, reliable, and valid measure for assessing severity and change of a wide range of fibromyalgia-related symptoms.
- Fibromyalgia is diagnosed when patients have widespread, chronic pain, at least 11 positive tender points, and no other medical illness to explain symptoms.

Keywords Abuse · Alexithymia · Tender point count · Tender point score · Psychological distress · Screening tools

Case: Helen H. is a frustrated 50-year-old CEO of a major company who has been treated for fibromyalgia for the past 8 years. "I just hate going to see the doctor. I'm there for fibromyalgia and instead of focusing on my pain complaints, he makes me answer questions and fill out questionnaires asking about my mood, sleep, bowel habits, and headaches. Why doesn't he just ask about my fibromyalgia?"

D.A. Marcus, A. Deodhar, *Fibromyalgia*, DOI 10.1007/978-1-4419-1609-9_4,
© Springer Science+Business Media, LLC 2011

Assessment of Fibromyalgia

Evaluating patients for fibromyalgia includes examining pain complaints, as well as other symptoms and conditions that occur frequently with fibromyalgia. Understanding the full symptom complex and impact from these symptoms will allow the clinician to best develop an effective treatment program. Furthermore, symptomatic improvement may initially occur with non-pain symptoms, such as sleep or mood disturbance. Not utilizing additional non-pain symptoms as markers of treatment outcome may result in failure identifying early treatment success and abandonment of treatments that might have eventually improved both pain and non-pain symptoms.

A useful fibromyalgia screening tool is the London Fibromyalgia Epidemiology Study Screening Questionnaire (Box 1) [1]. Sensitivity and specificity of the 4-item pain criteria alone are, respectively, 100 and 53%, with a test–retest reliability of 100% among those who screen negative and a positive predictive value of 57%. This tool has been successfully used to screen for fibromyalgia in both general population and patient samples [2, 3].

Box 1 The London Fibromyalgia Epidemiology Study Screening Questionnaire [1]

A. Pain criteria

In the past 3 months:
1. Have you had pain in muscles, bones, or joints, lasting at least 1 week?
2. Have you had pain in your shoulders, arms, or hands? On which side? Right, left, or both?
3. Have you had pain in your legs or feet? On which side? Right, left, or both?
4. Have you had pain in your neck, chest, or back?

Meeting the pain criteria requires "yes" responses to *all four* pain items, and either (1) both a right- and left-side positive response or (2) one both sides positive response

B. Fatigue criteria

1. Over the past 3 months, do you often felt tired or fatigued?
2. Does tiredness or fatigue significantly limit your activities?

Screening positive for chronic, debilitating fatigue requires a "yes" response to both fatigue items

A total positive response occurs when patients meet pain criteria alone or both pain and fatigue criteria

Pain Assessment

Diffuse pain may occur with a plethora of medical conditions (Box 2). Patients presenting with generalized pain complaints require a careful general medical history and examination to ensure the absence of potentially correctable or treatable medical conditions.

Box 2 Common Causes of Generalized Pain

- Ankylosing spondylitis
- Chronic hepatitis C
- Diabetes
- Fibromyalgia
- Hyperparathyroidism
- Hypothyroidism
- Lyme disease
- Metastatic cancer
- Multiple myeloma
- Osteoarthritis
- Osteomalacia
- Polymyalgia rheumatica
- Rheumatoid arthritis
- Sjögren's syndrome
- Systemic lupus erythematosus

Case: Lucia D. is a 68-year-old women treated with mastectomy for breast cancer. Five years previously, she was treated with tamoxifen after a breast biopsy revealed positive estrogen receptors. Two months later, she underwent mastectomy and continued tamoxifen. "Within the first 3 months on tamoxifen, I became increasingly aware of some generalized muscle and small joint discomfort with morning stiffness. And I became very fatigued after exercise. I also noticed generalized tenderness to touch of all my extremities and shoulders. At this point, I was diagnosed with fibromyalgia. After 4 years, my oncologist deemed I was cancer free and discontinued the tamoxifen. Over the next several months, generalized musculoskeletal discomfort and related symptoms abated." This case highlights the importance of ensuring fibromyalgia-like symptoms are not related to another condition. Interestingly, there are case reports of the development of fibromyalgia symptoms shortly after tamoxifen therapy was initiated, similar to Lucia' story [4]. Furthermore, raloxifene has been shown to reduce pain, tender points, and sleep disturbance in menopausal women with fibromyalgia [5].

(a)

Patients mark their pain severity on a 100 mm line. Pain severity is measured in mm from zero (no pain) to 100 mm (worst pain imaginable).

Mark your pain severity along this line:

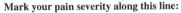

No pain ◆————————————————————◆ Worst pain imaginable

(b)

Patients rate pain severity from 0 (no pain) to 10 (unbearable pain).

Circle the number that indicates your pain severity:

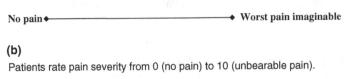

0	1	2	3	4	5	6	7	8	9	**10**
No Pain										Unbearable pain

(c)

Patients choose descriptors about pain from none – mild – moderate – severe.

Circle the term that indicates your pain severity:

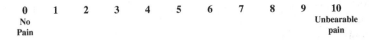

None   -   **Mild** -   **Moderate**   -   **Severe**

Fig. 1 Pain severity assessment measures: (**a**) Visual Analogue Scale; (**b**) Numeric Rating Scale; (**c**) Descriptive Scale

Pain severity can be quantified using a Visual Analogue Scale, Numeric Rating Scale, or Descriptive Scale (Fig. 1). In clinical practice, the Numeric Rating Scale is usually the easiest for patients to understand and doctors to quickly interpret. Numeric pain ratings of 5 or higher correlate with substantial pain-related interference and disability, with scores ≥5 signifying moderate pain and interference and scores ≥7–8 severe pain and interference [6].

Part of the physical examination of fibromyalgia is a tender point examination, an easy-to-perform bedside assessment. This examination catalogues the tenderness of 18 prespecified areas exposed to 4 kg pressure (Fig. 2). Pressing with the thumb results in approximately 4 kg of pressure when the nail bed blanches. Interestingly, digital palpation more effectively discriminates fibromyalgia patients than dolorimeter testing, making testing at the bedside easy [7]. Severity with pressing each point is assessed using a scale from 0 (no pain or pressure only) to 10 (excruciating pain). Higher scores reported for tender points correlate with greater levels of disability [8]. A diagnosis of fibromyalgia requires 11 positive points out of a possible 18 tested tender points. The tender point score will range from 0 to a maximum of 180. These measures are helpful for both diagnosis and as treatment outcome markers.

Practical pointer

Tender point count is the number of painful tender points. *Tender point score* is the sum of all recorded scores.

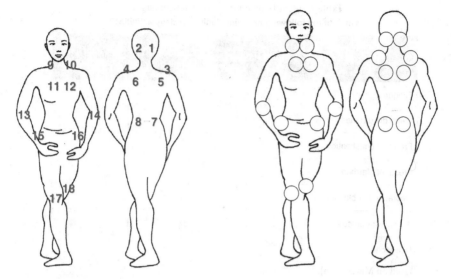

Fig. 2 Fibromyalgia tender point examination (reprinted from Marcus [16]). Test each labeled spot by exerting 4 kg of pressure with the thumb (watch for the nail bed to blanch). Record pain severity at each spot in the circles from 0 (none) to 10 (excruciating). Determine the tender point count (number of painful tender points scored >0) and tender point score (sum of all recorded scores)

Disability may be monitored using the Fibromyalgia Impact Questionnaire (FIQ; copy provided in the chapter "Clinical Handouts") [9]. This questionnaire assesses disability related to daily activities and work, as well as impact from pain, fatigue, and psychological distress. Patients can complete this self-administered questionnaire in about 5 min, making completion during typical clinic visits feasible. A 14% change in FIQ total score has been determined to represent a clinically relevant change [10].

> **Practical pointer**
>
> Self-administered questionnaires, like the Fibromyalgia Impact Questionnaire or FIQ, are easy and quick for patients to complete and serve as good measures of disability.

Assessment of Treatable Co-morbid Symptoms

Identifying treatable co-morbid symptoms can help clarify the most important treatment targets. Table 1 can be completed by patients to help determine which symptoms should be the focus of treatment.

Table 1 Identifying co-morbid treatment targets
Which of the following problems limit your daily activities?

Problem	Not a problem	Problem occurs but does NOT limit daily routine	Problem limits daily routine
Fatigue			
Sleep disturbance			
Frequent constipation			
Frequent diarrhea			
Depressed or blue mood			
Anxiety or nervousness			
Headache			

Based on Marcus [16].

Psychological Distress Screening

Psychological distress is common in patients with fibromyalgia. For example, a general population survey reported an annual prevalence of major depression in 22% of individuals with fibromyalgia vs. 7% without fibromyalgia [11]. In an interesting study, a general population sample was screened for the presence of chronic (>3 months duration) widespread pain [12]. Individuals with widespread pain were then evaluated with a tender point examination to identify if they met criteria for fibromyalgia. In this sample, fibromyalgia was diagnosed in 56% of individuals with chronic widespread pain. Psychological distress was higher among those with fibromyalgia, with significantly higher scores among those individuals with fibromyalgia on scales for depression (mean Beck Depression Inventory 12.3 ± 8.0 with fibromyalgia vs. 8.9 ± 5.9 without, $P=0.02$) and anxiety (mean Beck Anxiety Inventory 13.2 ± 9.7 with vs. 9.3 ± 7.0 without, $P=0.01$). The prevalence of depression is shown in Fig. 3.

All patients with fibromyalgia should be screened for depression and anxiety because of the high prevalence of mood disturbance with fibromyalgia. Many patients are reluctant to discuss psychological symptoms with their treating clinicians, for fear of being labeled as a psychiatric patient, with all fibromyalgia symptoms attributed to emotional problems. Also, unless symptoms are severe, many patients do not recognize symptoms of anxiety or depression. This may be especially common in fibromyalgia patients who also may experience alexithymia, a lack of emotional awareness or difficulty identifying feelings. In a recent survey of fibromyalgia patients, 19% were identified as alexithymic [13]. Interestingly, pain thresholds were similar for fibromyalgia patients with or without alexithymia, but pain tolerance was lower among those with alexithymia. Failure to readily identify psychological distress can lead patients to fail to seek necessary treatment. These

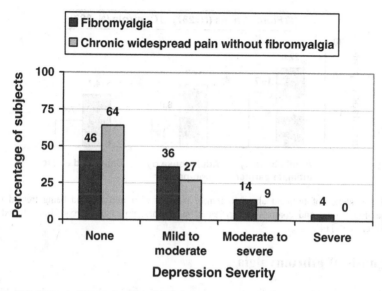

Fig. 3 Comparison of psychological distress among individuals with chronic widespread pain with and without fibromyalgia (based on Cöster et al. [12])

patients may mistakenly attribute their mood or anxiety symptoms to consequences of suffering from chronic pain and incorrectly assume that these symptoms will resolve spontaneously once the pain severity has improved. Untreated psychological distress can substantially add to the disability of fibromyalgia and reduce patients' ability to be motivated to participate and comply with prescribed treatment.

Practical pointer

Fibromyalgia patients should be routinely screened for depression and anxiety because of a high prevalence of mood disorders and because a substantial number also experience alexithymia – a difficulty in recognizing psychological distress.

Abuse occurs in a substantial number of fibromyalgia patients. In a comparison of frequent abuse in female patients seeing a rheumatologist for fibromyalgia or an ears, nose, and throat doctor for another condition, the odds ratios showed a higher likelihood among fibromyalgia patients of abuse as an adult by someone other than an intimate partner (odds ratio=2.20, 95% confidence interval 1.20–4.01) and childhood abuse (1.96, 1.03–3.74) [14] (see Fig. 4). Abuse as an adult by an intimate partner was not significantly higher among fibromyalgia patients (odds ratio=1.51, 95% confidence interval 0.93–2.44). Fibromyalgia patients, therefore, should also be directly asked if they have been or currently are victims of abuse.

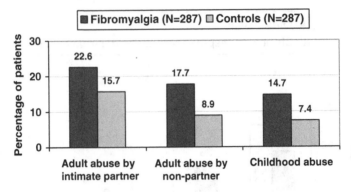

Fig. 4 Prevalence of frequent abuse in female patients with fibromyalgia being treated in a rheumatology clinic and controls being treated in an ears, nose, and throat clinic (based on Ruiz-Pérez et al. [14])

Diagnosis of Fibromyalgia

The diagnosis of fibromyalgia requires documentation of widespread pain and 11 of 18 painful tender points (Box 3), using a standardized tender point examination (see recording sheet in the chapter "Clinical Handouts"). Both tender point count and score should be recorded as baseline symptom severity measures to help document the diagnosis of fibromyalgia and to provide measures to use to monitor progress.

Box 3 Fibromyalgia Diagnostic Criteria (Based on American College of Rheumatology Criteria [7])

- Widespread body pain
  - Pain on both left and right sides of the body
  - Pain above and below the waist
  - Axial pain present
- Pain persisting ≥3 months
- ≥11 of 18 tender points painful to 4 kg pressure

Practical pointer

Fibromyalgia is diagnosed when:

- Pain has lasted for at least 3 months
- Pain is widespread
- At least 11 tender points are painful to pressure
- No other medical illness explains symptoms

At the time of diagnosis the following measures should be recorded and documented in the chart:

- Tender point count
- Tender point score
- Average pain severity (0=no pain, 10=excruciating and disabling pain)
- Average number of hours of nighttime sleep
- The presence and severity (none – mild – moderate – severe) of any of the following:

  - Disability for work or household chores
  - Disability for leisure, family, or social activities
  - Sleep disturbance
  - Bowel problems
  - Troublesome headaches
  - Excess weight
  - Depression or anxiety

A sample recording log is provided in the chapter "Clinical Handouts".

The FibroFatigue Scale was developed to assess a variety of common fibromyalgia symptoms [15]. The FibroFatigue Scale is a reliable and valid measure for assessing symptom severity and monitoring change during treatment (Table 2). This tool evaluates severity of a wide range of possible fibromyalgia-related symptoms.

Table 2 FibroFatigue Scale

The following symptoms are rated by a healthcare provider after asking general questions during a clinical interview

Symptom	Rate symptom severity 0=no or minimal symptoms 6=severe and disabling symptoms						
	0	1	2	3	4	5	6
Aches and pains							
Muscular tension							
Fatigue							
Concentration difficulties							
Failing memory							
Irritability							
Sadness							
Sleep disturbances							
Autonomic disturbances							
Irritable bowel							
Headache							
Subjective experience of infection							

Adapted from [15].

Summary

- The fibromyalgia assessment includes evaluating patients for a variety of pain and non-pain symptoms.
- The tender point examination is a necessary evaluation for diagnosing fibromyalgia. Monitoring tender point count and score can help evaluate treatment response.
- All fibromyalgia patients should be screened for co-morbid depression and anxiety because mood disturbance occurs commonly and fibromyalgia patients may also experience alexithymia, a lack of emotional awareness or difficulty identifying feelings.
- Reliable and validated tools, like the FibroFatigue Scale Questionnaire, can be used to document severity of a wide range of fibromyalgia-related symptoms and offer a tool for monitoring treatment progress.
- Fibromyalgia is diagnosed when patients have widespread, chronic pain, at least 11 positive tender points, and no other medical illness(es) to explain symptoms.

References

1. White KP, Speechley M, Harth M, Ostbye T. Testing an instrument to screen for fibromyalgia syndrome in general population studies: the London Fibromyalgia Epidemiology Study Screening Questionnaire. J Rheumatol. 1999;26:880–4.
2. White KP, Thompson J. Fibromyalgia syndrome in an Amish community: a controlled study to determine disease and symptom prevalence. J Rheumatol. 2003;30:1835–40.
3. Bannwarth B, Blotman F, Roué-Le Lay K, et al. Fibromyalgia syndrome in the general population of France: a prevalence study. Joint Bone Spine. 2009;76:184–7.
4. Warner E, Keshavjee A, Shupak R, Bellini A. Rheumatic symptoms following adjunctive therapy for breast cancer. Am J Clin Oncol. 1997;20:322–6.
5. Sadreddini S, Molaeefard M, Noshad H, Ardalan M, Asadi A. Efficacy of raloxifen in treatment of fibromyalgia in menopausal women. Eur J Intern Med. 2008;19:350–5.
6. Zelman DC, Hoffman DL, Seifeldin R, Dukes EM. Development of a metric for a day of manageable pain control: derivation of pain severity cut-points for low back pain and osteoarthritis. Pain. 2003;106:35–42.
7. Wolfe F, Smythe HA, Yunus MB, et al. The American College of Rheumatology 1990 criteria for the classification of fibromyalgia: report of the Multicenter Criteria Committee. Arthritis Rheum. 1990;33:160–72.
8. Lundberg G, Gerdle B. Tender point scores and their relations to signs of mobility, symptoms, and disability in female home care personnel and the prevalence of fibromyalgia. J Rheumatol. 2002;29:603–13.
9. Burckhardt CS, Clark SR, Bennett RM. The fibromyalgia impact questionnaire: development and validation. J Rheumatol. 1991;18:728–33.
10. Bennett RM, Bushmakin AG, Cappelleri JC, Zlateva G, Sadosky AB. Minimal clinically important difference in the Fibromyalgia Impact Questionnaire. J Rheumatol. 2009;36: 1304–11.
11. Kassam A, Patten SB. Major depression, fibromyalgia and labour force participation: a population-based cross-sectional study. BMC Musculoskel Disord. 2006;7:4.
12. Cöster L, Kendall S, Gerdle B, et al. Chronic widespread musculoskeletal pain – a comparison of those who meet criteria for fibromyalgia and those who do not. Eur J Pain. 2008;12: 600–10.

13. Huber A, Suman AL, Biasi G, Carli G. Alexithymia in fibromyalgia syndrome: associations with ongoing pain, experimental pain sensitivity and illness behavior. J Psychosom Res. 2009;66:425–33.
14. Ruiz-Pérez I, Palazaola-Castaño J, Càliz-Càliz R, et al. Risk factors for fibromyalgia: the role of violence against women. Clin Rheumatol. 2009;28:777–86.
15. Zachrisson O, Regland B, Jahreskog M, Kron M, Gottfires CG. A rating scale for fibromyalgia and chronic fatigue syndrome (the FibroFatigue scale). J Psychosom Res. 2002;52:501–9.
16. Marcus DA. Chronic pain. A primary care guide to practical management. Totowa, NJ: Humana Press; 2005.

Part II
Common Co-morbidities and Fibromyalgia

Headache

Key Chapter Points

- Three in every four fibromyalgia patients have troublesome headaches.
- Migraine can be divided into four phases: prodrome, aura, headache phase, and postdrome.
- Features of migraine prodrome and postdrome may mimic fibromyalgia symptoms, resulting in failure of patients to identify migraine.
- Healthy lifestyle changes, including regulation of eating and sleeping schedules, avoiding nicotine, and regular aerobic exercise, may reduce symptoms of recurring headaches and fibromyalgia.
- Infrequent, disabling headaches may be effectively treated with analgesics, triptans, or dihydroergotamine.
- Antidepressants and neuromodulating antiepileptics are first-line medications for headache prevention in patients with frequent attacks (regularly occurring >3 days per week).

Keywords Allodynia · Aura · Headache · Prodrome · Postdrome · Triptan

Case: Lisa is a 27-year-old legal secretary and mother of three who has been treated for fibromyalgia for the past 4 years. She comes to the office tearful that she was given a warning notice from work due to frequent absences over the last several months. "Ever since my last baby was born, I've been more stressed and getting less sleep and exercise and my pain just gets unbearable at times. I know it's just my fibromyalgia, but some days I'm feel so fatigued and out of it and just can't concentrate. Once that happens, the next day everything seems to bother me. I'm nauseated and just need to go to bed and I'm useless in the office." On further evaluation, the symptoms occurring on the days of work absence included a throbbing headache with sensitivity to noises, lights, and odors along with nausea. She was diagnosed with co-morbid migraine and these disabling migraine episodes were well managed with triptans, eliminating most cases of work absence.

D.A. Marcus, A. Deodhar, *Fibromyalgia*, DOI 10.1007/978-1-4419-1609-9_5,
© Springer Science+Business Media, LLC 2011

Co-morbidity has been demonstrated between fibromyalgia and headache in studies evaluating headache in patients with a primary complaint of fibromyalgia and migraine. In a survey of 100 treatment-seeking fibromyalgia patients, troublesome headache was reported by 76% of patients [1]. Migraine and tension-type headaches were the most commonly reported individual headaches (Fig. 1). Interestingly, although none of these patients was actively seeking treatment for headache, 80% rated the impact from their headaches as severe. Studies have also evaluated the prevalence of fibromyalgia in patients with a primary migraine diagnosis [2, 3]. These studies likewise showed co-morbidity between migraine and fibromyalgia, with this link stronger in patients with frequent migraine attacks (called chronic migraine) (Fig. 2).

Practical pointer

Nearly half of fibromyaglia patients have migraine. One in three fibromyalgia patients has tension-type headache.

Fig. 1 Prevalence of troublesome headache in fibromyalgia patients (based on Marcus et al. [1])

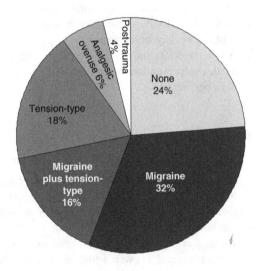

Pathophysiology of Headache and Fibromyalgia

Most studies evaluating the pathogenesis of chronic headaches have focused on migraine. Changes in activity in the pons are believed to be essential to the development of migraine, with pontine dysfunction acting as an important migraine

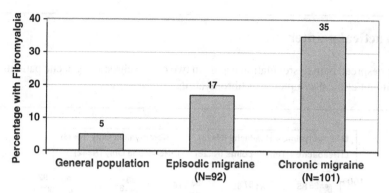

Fig. 2 Prevalence of fibromyalgia in migraine sufferers (based on Ifergane et al. [2] and Peres et al. [3]). Migraine can be divided based on frequency of attacks. When attacks typically occur <15 days per month, they are considered *episodic*; attacks generally occurring ≥15 days per month are considered *chronic*

generator [4]. The role of the pons in the development of migraine was supported by a case report describing migraine in a patient with a pontine vascular malformation [5]. More recently, a physiological link between the abnormal central pain processing in the pons and the development of migraine plus fibromyalgia was suggested by an interesting case report of a 42-year-old woman who developed migraine-like headaches and 14 positive tender points 2 months after recovering from a pontine hemorrhage [6].

Neurotransmitter abnormalities and central sensitization are common to both chronic headaches and fibromyalgia. For example, changes in serotonin, norepinephrine, and dopamine have been identified as important factors for headache and fibromyalgia, with effective treatments targeting corrections in these neurotransmitter imbalances. Calcitonin gene-related peptide (CGRP) is also important in the pathophysiology of headache, resulting in increased vasodilation and transmission of pain messages [7]. CGRP changes in fibromyalgia have been inconsistently reported. Widespread dysregulation of pain modulation has been identified in chronic headache patients, providing another physiological link with fibromyalgia [8]. In one study, patients seeking treatment for widespread pain from fibromyalgia ($N = 66$) or localized pain only (chronic headache, $N = 70$) were evaluated with a fibromyalgia tender point examination [8]. By definition, ≥11 tender points were expected to be present in the fibromyalgia patients. Interestingly, 40% of the chronic headache patients also had ≥11 positive tender points. Despite reports of pain localized to the head, the location of positive tender points in the headache patients was not focused around the head, neck, and shoulder girdle. The distribution of positive tender points was similarly widespread in patients with either a clinical diagnosis of headache or fibromyalgia (Fig. 3). Severity of pain perceived during the tender point testing was also similar for fibromyalgia and headache patients, further supporting analogous widespread pain dysfunction in both patient groups.

Practical pointer

Widespread pain dysregulation occurs in two of five chronic headache patients without clinical symptoms of fibromyalgia.

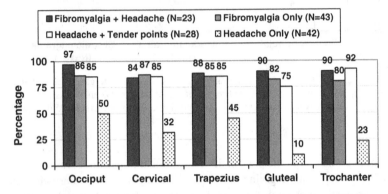

Fig. 3 Pain dysregulation in fibromyalgia and headache (based on Okifuji et al. [8]). Among the fibromyalgia patients, 35% reported chronic headaches. None of the headache patients reported widespread or diffuse pain. Among the headache patients, 40% had ≥11 positive tender points on their examination. The remaining 60% of headache patients were termed "headache only"

Evaluation and Diagnosis

All patients describing headache should be evaluated with a detailed history and medical and neurological examinations to ensure the absence of a secondary headache from another condition (Box 1). Common headaches are distinguished based on symptom characteristics (Table 1). Most chronic headaches evaluated in

Box 1 Clinical Features Suggesting a Work-Up for Secondary Headache May Be Necessary

- Patient ≥50 years old
- Significant change in headache quality or pattern within the last 2 years
- Pain in the posterior head or neck
- Additional medical symptoms
- Additional neurological symptoms
- Abnormal physical or neurological findings

Table 1 Diagnostic features of common headaches

Headache type	General description	Typical untreated headache episode duration in adults	Associated features
Primary headaches			
Migraine	Intermittent, recurring, disabling headache	4–24 h	Desire to isolate self Sensitivity to lights, noises, and odors Nausea or vomiting Temporary aura symptoms occur before or with migraine in about one in five migraine sufferers, most commonly visual hallucinations, like colored balls, sparkling lights, zigzag lines, or blind spots
Tension type	Mild, non-disabling headache that may be intermittent or constant	30 min to several days	Tenderness of muscles over the head and neck
Cluster	Excruciating, orbital or periorbital pain	30 min–2 h	Attacks associated with increased activity and often a desire to pace, shower, smoke, or bang head. Autonomic changes (rhinorrhea and lacrimation) are pronounced, but rarely noticed by patients
Secondary headaches			
Post-trauma	Headache often severe and disabling during the first 2 weeks after mild head injury with concussion. Over time, headache becomes milder	Initially, often constant with frequency of headaches and duration of attacks diminishing over time	Headache begins within 1 week of a concussion. May be associated with other features of post-concussion syndrome (mood disturbance, memory/concentration problems, dizziness, tinnitus); recovery is delayed in patients with pre-morbid migraine [48]
Medication overuse	Mild, non-disabling headache	Constant with fluctuating severity throughout the day	Prescription and/or over-the-counter acute medications are regularly used >3 days per week for at least 6 weeks

Table 2 Diagnosis of outpatient headache patients (based on Felício et al. [9])

Headache category	Diagnosis	Percentage
Primary headaches		
	All primary diagnoses	84
	Migraine	52
	Tension type	24
	Cluster	4
	Other	4
Secondary headaches		
	All secondary diagnoses	16
	Disorder of cranium, sinuses, teeth, or other cranial or facial structures	3
	Neuralgia	3
	Post-trauma	1
	Substance or its withdrawal	1
	Homeostasis disorder	1
	Vascular disorder	<1
	Non-vascular intracranial disorder	<1
	Infection	<1
	Psychiatric disorder	<1
	Other	6

outpatients are caused by primary headache disorders (like migraine, tension-type, and cluster headaches). A recent study cataloging headache diagnoses among outpatients referred to a tertiary headache center identified a minority of patients with secondary headaches (Table 2) [9].

Practical pointer

Outpatients seeking treatment for chronically recurring headaches are most commonly diagnosed with migraine.

A diagnostic algorithm can help distinguish headache types (Fig. 4). Patients using excessive amounts of acute headache medication (e.g., analgesics or triptans) may experience a headache worsening, called analgesic overuse headache. Analgesic overuse headache should be considered in patients regularly using acute headache medication more than 3 days per week for at least 6 weeks. Analgesic overuse headache is usually a mild, daily, non-disabling headache. In most cases, analgesic overuse headache improves several weeks to months after discontinuing the overused medication. Medication detoxification results in substantial headache improvement after 2 months in three in every four patients overusing acute headache

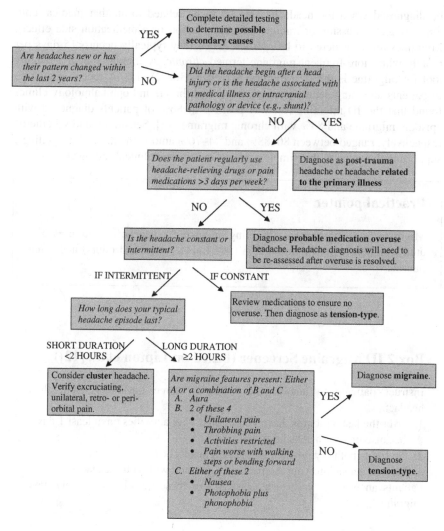

Fig. 4 Headache diagnostic algorithm (reproduced with permission from Marcus [45])

medication [10]. Tension-type headache is a mild, constant or intermittent, non-disabling headache in patients without medication overuse. Cluster headache is a relatively rare headache, characterized by typically nocturnal episodes of brief, excruciating orbital or periorbital pain.

Migraine

Migraine is diagnosed in patients with chronic, recurring, intermittent, disabling headaches who have characteristic associated symptoms [11]. Migraine should not be diagnosed when the headache appears to be related to another medical condition (e.g., concussion or trauma, infection, tumor, or a medication side effect). Migraines are considered to be *episodic* when they typically occur <15 days per month, with more frequent migraine termed *chronic*. A simple clinical screening tool for migraine is the ID Migraine Screener (Box 2) [12]. A recent evaluation of patients attending neurology, ears, nose, and throat, and ophthalmology clinics found that the ID migraine test was positive in 86% of patients diagnosed with episodic migraine and 83% with chronic migraine [13]. Sensitivity and specificity, respectively, ranged between 80–88% and 74–76% among the three clinic settings, supporting the value of this simple screener in different clinical settings.

Practical pointer

Migraine is an intermittent, disabling, recurring headache condition associated with sensitivity to stimulation (like lights, noise, and odors) and often nausea.

Box 2 ID Migraine Screener (based on Lipton et al. [12])

Instruct patients to answer the following three questions about their headaches:
1. Over the last 3 months, have you limited your activities on at least 1 day because of your headaches?
2. Do lights bother you when you have a headache?
3. Do you get sick to your stomach or nauseated with your headache?
Patients answering "yes" to at least two of these questions probably have migraine

---

Migraine attacks can be divided into four phases:

- Prodrome
- Aura
- Headache symptoms
- Postdrome

Features of each phase are described in Table 3. Due to the similarity of many of these symptoms with fibromyalgia (e.g., pain, fatigue, irritability, poor concentration), fibromyalgia patients may fail to link prodrome and postdrome symptoms to migraine and inadvertently attribute them to fibromyalgia. Identifying the

Table 3 Phases of migraine

Phase	Percentage of migraine patients experiencing	Features	Timing
Prodrome	30	Irritability, neck pain, food cravings, yawning, mood changes, diarrhea, constipation, loss of appetite, poor concentration, dizziness, fatigue	12–24 h before headache phase
Aura	15–20	Visual changes (blind spots, colored balls, shimmering lights, zigzag lines), unilateral numbness or weakness, confusion	5–60 min before headache phase or during the headache phase
Headache phase	Nearly 100	Throbbing pain, disability, nausea, sensitivity to noises, lights, and odors	8–24 h
Postdrome	70	Hung-over feeling, fatigue, poor concentration, loss of appetite, low-grade discomfort	12–24 h after headache phase

prodrome can be particularly helpful because acute treatment during the prodrome can reduce the severity of the headache phase [14]. Likewise, administering effective acute migraine treatment during the aura phase can also prevent progression of the migraine into the painful headache phase [15].

Practical pointer

Pain, irritability, and poor concentration occur commonly before and after migraine attacks. These migraine features may be confused with fibromyalgia symptom flares.

Treatment

Similar non-medication treatments that may help reduce fibromyalgia symptoms may likewise improve migraine and tension-type headaches, although most studies have focused on migraine (Table 4). The most effective non-medication treatments for migraine are stress management, relaxation, and biofeedback, which are each as effective as standard headache prevention medications. Non-medication treatments that may reduce cluster headache attacks include avoidance of alcohol and nicotine.

Table 4 Non-medication treatments for migraine and tension type

Treatment	Recommendations
Diet [46–48, 50, 51]	Avoid fasting. Individual foods are triggers for only about 30% of migraine sufferers
Sleeping [52]	Sleeping >6 and up to 8 h nightly
Nicotine [53, 54]	Discontinue smoking and other use of nicotine. Migraine risk as well as headache frequency and severity have been linked to smoking
Stress management [52–54, 56, 57]	Stress is the number 1 headache trigger. Stress management effectively reduces headaches by about 60%, with superior benefits to prevention medication in one study
Relaxation with or without biofeedback [55–57, 59, 60]	About 50–80% of patients motivated to learn these techniques experience relief. Similar efficacy to standard migraine prevention medication
Aerobic exercise [61]	Aerobic exercise three times weekly reduced migraine severity by 44% and duration by 36%

Headache medications are divided into acute and preventive therapies, with similar treatments effective for both migraine and tension-type headaches. Acute therapies are designed to be used infrequently, while preventive therapies are used daily to help reduce frequent headaches. Ideally, preventive therapies used in patients with co-morbid migraine or tension-type headaches and fibromyalgia would treat both pain conditions (Fig. 5). Combining both medication and non-medication therapy (e.g., relaxation and biofeedback) maximizes headache improvement [16].

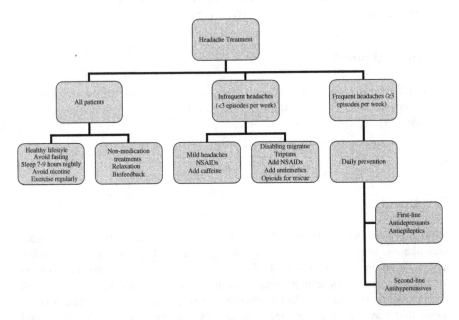

Fig. 5 Treatment of co-morbid migraine and tension-type headache

Acute Treatment for Migraine and Tension-Type Headache

Acute headache treatment should be limited to ≤3 days per week to avoid the risk for developing medication overuse headaches. Patients regularly using acute medications more frequently will need to have overused medications tapered and discontinued. Persistent frequent headaches should be managed with prevention therapy.

Mild-moderate severity headaches may be well managed with analgesics. Aspirin and nonsteroidal anti-inflammatory drugs are more effective than acetaminophen and opioids for reducing mild-moderate severity headache. Adding caffeine 100 mg to acute analgesics improves the number of people getting headache relief by 1.5 times [17]. Severe migraine attacks should be treated with a triptan or dihydroergotamine (Table 5). Both triptans and dihydroergotamine have vasoconstrictive properties and should not be used in patients with cardiovascular disease. Most patients will respond to at least one of the three triptan trials, so this class of medications should not be abandoned due to poor response to one or two triptans [18]. Migraine episodes with more severe symptoms are less likely to respond to treatment [19]; therefore, patients should treat several migraine episodes with a single triptan before abandoning that therapy as ineffective. Combining a triptan with an analgesic (e.g., triptan plus nonsteroidal anti-inflammatory drug) may increase the duration of headache relief [20].

Table 5 Selection of acute migraine treatment

Headache feature	Preferred medication category	Individual choices
Headache reaches peak severity quickly	Fast-acting injectable or intranasal triptan	Injectable or intranasal sumatriptan Intranasal zolmitriptan
Typical disabling migraine	Fast-acting oral triptan	Rizatriptan, eletriptan, zolmitriptan, sumatriptan, or almotriptan
Migraine usually lasts >24 h	Medication with better sustained relief	Dihydroergotamine
Migraine symptoms recur after triptan	Medication with better sustained relief	Fast-acting triptan PLUS nonsteroidal anti-inflammatory drug or dihydroergotamine
Poor tolerability of triptans	Triptan with fewer side effects	Naratriptan or frovatriptan
Desire for convenient formulation	Orally disintegrating tablets that do not require water	Orally disintegrating rizatriptan or zolmitriptan

Promising emerging therapies for migraine include CGRP-antagonists and intranasal carbon dioxide. Promising results have been published with an intravenous CGRP-antagonist BIBN4096BS and an oral preparation telecagepant [21].

Intravenous BIBN4096BS 2.5 mg produced 2-h headache relief in 66% vs. 27% with placebo. Efficacy with telecagepant 300 mg is similar to that achieved with zolmitriptan or rizatriptan [22, 23]. CGRP receptor antagonists lack direct vasoconstrictor properties and may offer an effective alternative for patients unable to use triptans because of cardiovascular risk factors or those failing to achieve adequate response from acute triptan therapy. Carbon dioxide may also have a role as acute headache treatment. Carbon dioxide inhibits sensory nerve activation and CGRP secretion, suggesting possible mechanisms for relieving acute headaches [24]. Early phase II clinical trial data have shown the effectiveness of 100% CO_2 delivered intranasally at a flow rate of 10 mL/s [25].

Migraines are most effectively treated with acute therapy when that therapy begins prior to the development of central sensitization. Studies by Rami Burstein and colleagues show that cutaneous allodynia (a perception of touch stimuli as painful) is an effective marker of central sensitization, with acute treatment efficacy reduced after cutaneous allodynia is established [26]. Clinical symptoms of allodynia are shown in Table 6. Patients should be instructed to monitor their headaches to identify when symptoms of allodynia typically take place so they can time acute treatment administration to occur prior to the onset of these symptoms to maximize successful migraine resolution.

Practical pointer

Acute migraine medications treat individual headache episodes and should be limited to no more than 3 days per week on a regular basis. Ideally, acute medications are administered before symptoms of cutaneous allodynia occur.

Patients with pronounced nausea with migraine may benefit from the addition of anti-emetics to their acute migraine treatment. Anti-emetics provide helpful adjunctive treatment for headache associated with nausea rather than migraine monotherapy [27, 28, 29]. In general, anti-emetics are more effective than metoclopramide.

Table 6 Cutaneous allodynia in migraine

Area of allodynia	Typical patient symptoms
Scalp sensitivity	Brushing or touching hair is painful. Patients often report "my hair hurts"
Facial sensitivity	Wearing glasses or earrings is painful. Shaving hurts
Body sensitivity	Clothing feels extra-tight. Patients prefer to avoid being touched.

Prevention Treatment for Frequent Migraine or Tension-Type Headache

The most effective prevention medications include antidepressants (especially tricyclics as first-line treatment), antiepileptics (topiramate and valproate as first-line treatment and gabapentin as second-line treatment), and antihypertensives (beta-blockers as first-line treatment and calcium channel blockers as second-line treatment). In general, first-line preventive medications result in about a 50–65% reduction in headache activity. Tonabersat is a promising new therapy being tested as a migraine prevention therapy. Tonabersat is a gap junction blocker, inhibiting cortical spreading depression and its consequences in migraine pathogenesis. In a double-blind, placebo-controlled trial, patients with active migraine were treated with tonabersat initiated at 20 mg daily for 2 weeks and increased to 40 mg daily for an additional 10 weeks [30]. Headache reduction by ≥50% occurred in 62% treated with tonabersat vs. 45% with placebo.

Selection of an individual prevention therapy for a particular patient generally relies on utilizing drugs that will treat headache as well as co-morbid conditions, such as depression, anxiety, sleep disturbance, or hypertension. Fibromyalgia patients with co-morbid headache should likewise initially be treated with medications that may improve headache as well as fibromyalgia symptoms or other co-morbidities.

> **Practical pointer**
>
> Selection of prevention therapy should consider co-morbid conditions that might be additionally treated with the prevention medication.

Some antiepileptic and antidepressant drugs effectively reduce fibromyalgia symptoms and may additionally reduce migraine. Gamma-aminobutyric acid-mediated neuromodulating antiepileptic drugs offer effective prevention of migraine [31]. Although pregabalin has not been directly tested in migraine, it has been reported anecdotally to reduce migraines and may be worth trying in fibromyalgia to achieve reduction in both migraines and fibromyalgia symptoms [32]. Likewise, antidepressants, especially tricyclics are considered first-line treatment for migraine prevention. Duloxetine has shown modest benefit in migraine prevention, with a ≥50% improvement of migraine in 22% of patients treated with duloxetine 30–90 mg daily [33]. In an open-label trial of 30 patients with major depression and chronic headache, a >50% improvement of depression and >40% reduction in pain occurred in 67% of patients treated with duloxetine 60 mg daily [34]. Milnacipran has not been studied in migraine. If antiepileptics and antidepressants that also reduce fibromyalgia symptoms are not effective as migraine prevention in fibromyalgia patients, if may be worthwhile investigating more standard migraine prevention therapy.

Common medication-related side effects may be confused with fibromyalgia symptoms. Sedation and cognitive effects are frequent problematic side effects from headache prevention therapies. Furthermore, the Food and Drug Administration recently announced a warning about increased risk of suicide among patients using some antiepileptic drugs, including gabapentin, pregabalin, topiramate, and valproate [35]. Change in mood can also occur in patients treated with beta-blocker antihypertensive medications.

Injections and Alternative Treatments

Hyperalgesia of the neck and shoulder girdle muscles is common in patients with migraine or tension-type headaches [36]. Myofascial trigger points are characterized by contracted and tender muscles with discrete areas of focal tenderness; palpating these trigger points may refer pain to the head (Fig. 6). Trigger points in the temporalis muscle occur commonly in patients with tension-type headache [37]. In patients with a myofascial component to their headaches, treatment with postural correction, stretching, and range of motion exercises is often helpful. Trigger point

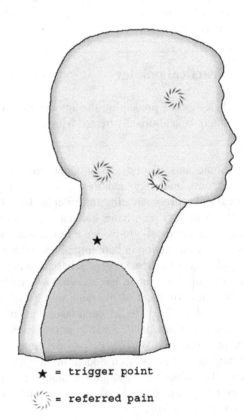

Fig. 6 Referral pattern for upper trazepius trigger points (reproduced with permission from Marcus [46])

★ = trigger point

⁝ = referred pain

injections with local anesthetic may also be helpful. A 22- to 25-gauge needle is inserted into the skin approximately 1 cm away from the trigger point, and then advanced to the trigger point. After verification of its placement outside of blood vessels, 0.1–0.2 mL of anesthetic is injected. This process is repeated at other areas within the trigger point until muscle spasm is reduced or 0.5–1.0 mL of anesthetic has been injected. Trigger points may also be treated using superficial dry needling, insertion of a solid thin needle (resembling an acupuncture needle) into trigger point with no anesthetic injection. In a small study, similar significant improvement in pain and range of motion occurred in patients with myofascial shoulder pain treated with either lidocaine trigger point injections ($N = 21$) or dry needling ($N = 18$) [38].

Occipital nerve blocks have also been shown to reduce headache activity in patients with frequent, recalcitrant headaches [39, 40]. The greater occipital nerve is located between the external occipital protuberance and the mastoid process, about 2 cm lateral to the external occipital protuberance (Fig. 7) [41]. In one series, 46% of unilateral greater occipital nerve blocks administered to migraine patients resulted in complete or partial pain [42]. Each block used a 3 mL mixture of 2% lidocaine and 80 mg of methylprednisolone. Most patients experienced complete relief for 7 days, with a mean duration of relief of 20 days. Partial response lasted for 20 days in most patients, with a mean duration of partial response of 45 days. Patients with pre-treatment tenderness over the greater occipital nerve were more likely to experience benefit from occipital nerve blocks.

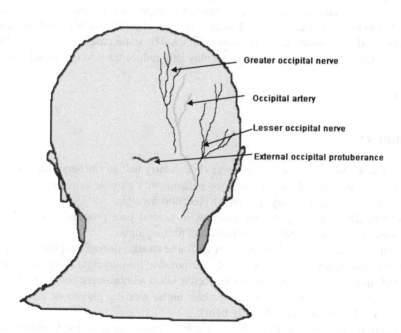

Fig. 7 Occipital nerve anatomy (reprinted with permission from Marcus and Bain [47])

Botulinum toxin type A is routinely used in cosmetic procedures to reduce facial lines and has been tested in multiple trials as a migraine preventive agent. A recent review evaluating the published efficacy of migraine preventive therapies determined that the available evidence does not support recommending botulinum toxin injections as an effective migraine prevention therapy [43].

In a recently published study, acupuncture was tested against sham acupuncture for the treatment of a single acute migraine attack [44]. Pain reduction was significant with both true and sham acupunctures. Two and four hours after treatment, pain reduction was significantly better with true acupuncture. At least partial pain relief occurred in >90% of patients in either group, although complete relief occurred in 41% with true acupuncture vs. 17% with sham acupuncture. Acupuncture has also been tested as a migraine preventive therapy. In general, studies consistently show no better result from patients randomized to receive real acupuncture vs. sham acupuncture [43].

Cluster Headache Treatment

Cluster headaches are primarily treated with prevention therapy, due to their severity and repetitive course. Furthermore, most acute therapies will not become effective during the course of these brief attacks. In general, cluster headaches are typically treated with preventive therapy for the expected duration of the cluster cycle, usually about 6 weeks. The most effective prevention therapies are verapamil and methysergide (no longer available in the United States). A short course of prednisone can also be used in patients with very severe attacks. In some cases, 100% O_2 delivered at 7 L/min for 10 min by face mask may help reduce the severity of individual attacks.

Summary

- Headache and fibromyalgia are co-morbid. Nearly half of fibromyalgia patients have migraine and about one in three patients with chronic migraine (frequent attacks occurring ≥15 days per month) has fibromyalgia.
- Abnormalities in the pons and changes in central pain processing have been linked to the development of migraine and fibromyalgia.
- Symptoms occurring before and after migraine attacks, during the prodrome and postdrome phases, may be incorrectly attributed to fibromyalgia symptom flares.
- Acute migraine treatments are most effective when administered before the development of cutaneous allodynia (e.g., hair hurts, wearing glasses or earrings is painful, clothing feels excessively tight).
- Antidepressants and neuromodulating antiepileptics are first-line treatment for headache prevention.

- Initial headache prevention medication selection in fibromyalgia patients should include medications proven to reduce fibromyalgia symptoms in addition to headache.
- Patients failing to benefit from fibromyalgia therapy may need to utilize standard first-line headache prevention, including tricyclic antidepressants, topiramate, valproate, and beta-blockers.

References

1. Marcus DA, Bernstein C, Rudy TE. Fibromyalgia and headache: an epidemiological study supporting migraine as part of the fibromyaglia syndrome. Clin Rheumatol. 2005;24:595–601.
2. Ifergane G, Buskila D, Simiseshvely N, Zeev K, Cohen H. Prevalence of fibromyalgia syndrome in migraine patients. Cephalalgia. 2006;26:451–6.
3. Peres MF, Young WB, Kaup AO, Zukerman E, Silberstein SD. Fibromyalgia is common in patients with transformed migraine. Neurology. 2001;57:1326–8.
4. Tajti J, Uddman R, Edvinsson L. Neuropeptide localization in the "migraine generator" region of the human brainstem. Cephalalgia. 2001;21:96–101.
5. Obermann M, Gizewski ER, Limmroth V, Diener HC, Katsarava Z. Symptomatic migraine and pontine vascular malformation: evidence for a key role of the brainstem in the pathophysiology of chronic migraine. Cephalalgia. 2006;26:763–6.
6. Ifergane G, Shelef I, Buskila D. Migraine and fibromyalgia developing after a pontine hemorrhage. Cephalalgia. 2007;27:191.
7. Panconesi A, Bartolozzi ML, Guidi L. Migraine pain: reflections against vasodilation. J Headache Pain. 2009;10:317–25.
8. Okifuji A, Turk DC, Marcus DA. Comparison of generalized and localized hyperalgesia in patients with recurrent headache and fibromyalgia. Psychosom Med. 1999;61:771–80.
9. Felício AC, Bischuette DB, dos Santos WC, et al. Epidemiology of primary and secondary headaches in a Brazilian tertiary-care center. Arq Neuropsiquiatr. 2006;64:41–4.
10. Rossi P, Di Lorenzo C, Faroni J, Cesarino F, Nappi G. Advice alone vs. structured detoxification programmes for medication overuse headache: a prospective, randomized, open-label trial in transformed migraine patients with low medical needs. Cephalalgia. 2006;26: 1097–105.
11. Headache Classification Subcommittee of the International Headache Society. The international classification of headache disorders, 2nd edn. Cephalalgia. 2004;24:1–160.
12. Lipton RB, Dodick D, Sadovsky R, et al. A self-administered screener for migraine in primary care: The ID Migraine validation study. Neurology. 2003;61:375–82.
13. Ertas M, Baykan B, Tuncel D, et al. A comparative ID migraine™ screener study in ophthalmology, ENT and neurology out-patient clinics. Cephalalgia. 2009;29:68–75.
14. Evans RW, Mannix LK. Triptans for migraine prodrome. Headache. 2002;42:83–4.
15. Aurora SK, Barrodale PM, McDonald SA, Jakubowski M, Burstein R. Revisiting the efficacy of sumatriptan therapy during the aura phase of migraine. Headache. 2009;49:1001–4.
16. Holroyd KA, France JL, Cordingley GE, et al. Enhancing the effectiveness of relaxation-thermal biofeedback training with propranolol hydrochloride. J Consult Clin Psychol. 1995;63:327–30.
17. Peroutka SJ, Lyon JA, Swarbrick J, Lipton RB, Kolodner K, Goldstein J. Efficacy of diclofenac sodium softgel 100 mg with or without caffeine 100 mg in migraine without aura: a randomized, double-blind, crossover study. Headache. 2004;44:136–41.
18. Mathew NT, Kailasam J, Gentry P, Chernyshev O. Treatment of nonresponders to oral sumatriptan with zolmitriptan and rizatriptan: a comparative open trial. Headache. 2000;40:464–5.
19. Diener HC, Dodick DW, Goadsby PJ, et al. Identification of negative predictors of pain-free response to triptans: analysis of the eletriptan database. Cephalalgia. 2007;28:35–40.

20. Krymchantowski AV, Barbosa JS. Rizatriptan combined with rofecoxib vs. rizatriptan for the acute treatment of migraine: an open label pilot study. Cephalalgia. 2002;22:309–12.

21. Salvatore CA, Hershey JC, Corcoran HA, et al. Pharmacological characterization of MK-0974 [N-[(3R,6S)-6-(2,3-difluorophenyl)-2-oxo-1-(2,2,2-trifluoroethyl)azepan-3-yl]-4-(2-oxo-2,3-dihydro-1H-imidazo[4,5-b]pyridin-1-yl)piperidine-1-carboxamide], a potent and orally active calcitonin gene-related peptide receptor antagonist for the treatment of migraine. J Pharmacol Exp Ther. 2008;324:416–21.

22. Ho TW, Ferrari MD, Dodick DW, et al. Efficacy and tolerability of MK-0974 (telcagepant), a new oral antagonist of calcitonin gene-related peptide receptor, compared with zolmitriptan for acute migraine: a randomised, placebo-controlled, parallel-treatment trial. Lancet. 2008;372:2115–23.

23. Ho TW, Mannix LK, Fan X, et al. Randomized controlled trial of an oral CGRP receptor antagonist, MK-0974, in acute treatment of migraine. Neurology. 2008;70:1304–12.

24. Vause C, Bowen E, Spierings E, Durham P. Effect of carbon dioxide on calcitonin gene-related peptide secretion from trigeminal neurons. Headache. 2007;47:1385–97.

25. Spierings G. Abortive treatment of migraine headache with non-inhaled, intranasal carbon dioxide: a randomized, double-blind, placebo-controlled, parallel-group study. Headache. 2005;45:809.

26. Burstein R, Levy D, Jakubowski M. Effects of sensitization of trigeminovascular neurons to triptan therapy during migraine. Rev Neurol. (Paris) 2005;161:658–60.

27. Jones J, Pack S, Chun E. Intramuscular prochlorperazine versus metoclopramide as single-agent therapy for the treatment of acute migraine headache. Ann Emerg Med. 1996;14:262–4.

28. Friedman BW, Esses D, Soloranzo C, et al. A randomized controlled trial of prochlorperazine versus metoclopramide for treatment of acute migraine. Ann Emerg Med. 2008;52:399–406.

29. Gruppo LQ. Intravenous Zofran for headache. J Emerg Med. 2006;31:228–9.

30. Goadsby PJ, Ferrari MD, Olesen J, Mills JG. Randomized, double-blind, placebo-controlled, proof-of-concept study of the cortical spreading depression inhibiting agent tonabersat in migraine prophylaxis. Cephalalgia. 2009;29:742–50.

31. Calabresi P, Galletti F, Rossi C, Sarchielli P, Cupini LM. Antiepileptic drugs in migraine: from clinical aspects to cellular mechanism. Trends Pharmacol Sci. 2008;28:188–95.

32. Masdrakis VG, Oulis P, Karakatsanis NA, et al. Remission of migraine attacks in a patient with depression who is taking pregabalin. Clin Neuropharmacol. 2008;31:238–40.

33. Taylor AP, Adelman JU, Freeman MC. Efficacy of duloxetine as a migraine prevention medication: possible predictors of response in a retrospective chart review. Headache. 2007;47:1200–3.

34. Volpe FM. An 8-week, open-label trial of duloxetine for comorbid major depressive disorder and chronic headache. J Clin Psychiatry. 2008:e1–6.

35. http://www.fda.gov/cder/drug/InfoSheets/HCP/antiepilepticsHCP.htm. Accessed February 2008.

36. Fernández-de-las-Peñas C, Madeleine P, Caminero AB, et al. Generalized neck-shoulder hyperalgesia in chronic tension-type headache and unilateral migraine assessed by pressure pain sensitivity topographical maps of the trapezius muscle. Cephalalgia, in press.

37. Fernández-de-las-Peñas C, Caminero AB, Madeleine P, et al. Multiple active myofascial trigger points and pressure pain sensitivity maps in the temporalis muscle are related in women with chronic tension type headache. Clin J Pain. 2009;25:506–12.

38. Ga H, Choi J, Park C, Yoon H. Acupuncture needling versus lidocaine injection of trigger points in myofascial pain syndrome in elderly patients – a randomized trial. Acupunct Med. 2007;25:130–6.

39. Ashkenazi A, Levin M. Greater occipital nerve block for migraine and other headaches: is it useful? Curr Pain Headache Rep. 2007;11:231–5.

40. Ashkenazi AA, Matro R, Shaw JW, Abbas MA, Silberstein SD. Greater occipital nerve block using local anesthetics alone or with triamcinolone for transformed migraine: a randomized comparative study. J Neurol Neurosurg Psychiatry. 2008;79:415–7.

41. Loukas M, El-Sedfy A, Tubbs RS, et al. Identification of greater occipital nerve landmarks for the treatment of occipital neuralgia. Folia Morph. 2006;65:337–42.
42. Afridi SK, Shields KG, Bhola R, Goadsby PJ. Greater occipital nerve injection in primary headache symptoms – prolonged effects from a single injection. Pain. 2006;122:126–9.
43. Schürks M, Diener H, Goadsby P. Update on the prophylaxis of migraine. Curr Treat Opt Neurol. 2008;10:20–9.
44. Li Y, Liang F, Yang X, et al. Acupuncture for treating acute attacks of migraine: a randomized controlled trial. Headache. 2009;49:805–16.
45. Marcus DA. Headache simplified. Nr Shrewsbury, UK: TFM Publishing; 2008.
46. Marcus DA. Chronic pain. A primary care guide to practical management, 2nd edn. Totowa, NJ: Humana Press; 2009.
47. Marcus DA, Bain, PA. Effective migraine treatment in pregnant and lactating women. New York, NY: Springer; 2009.
48. Lau B, Lovell MR, Collins MW, Pardini J. Neurocognitive and symptom predictors of recovery in high school athletes. Clin J Sport Med. 2009;19:216–21.
49. Medina JL, Diamond S. The role of diet in migraine. Headache. 1978;18:31–4.
50. Mosek A, Korczyn AD. Yom Kippur headache. Neurology. 1995;45:1953–5.
51. Topacoglu H, Karcioglu O, Yuruktumen A, et al. Impact of Ramadan on demographics and frequencies of disease-related visits in the emergency department. Int J Clin Pract. 2005;59:900–5.
52. Kelman L, Rains JC. Headache and sleep: examination of sleep patterns and complaints in a large clinical sample of migraineurs. Headache. 2005;45:904–10.
53. Hozawa A, Houston T, Steffes MW, et al. The association of cigarette smoking with self-reported disease before middle age: the Coronary Artery Risk Development in Young Adults (CARDIA) study. Pre Med. 2006;42:193–9.
54. Payne TJ, Stetson B, Stevens VM, Johnson CA, Penzien DB, Van Dorsten B. Impact of cigarette smoking on headache activity in headache patients. Headache. 1991;31:329–32.
55. Kohlenberg RT, Cahn T. Self-help treatment for migraine headaches: a controlled outcome study. Headache. 1981;21:196–200.
56. Mitchell KR, White RG. Control of migraine headache by behavioral self-management: a controlled case study. Headache. 1976;16:178–84.
57. Cordingley G, Holrody K, Pingel J, Jerome A, Nash J. Amitriptyline versus stress management therapy in the prophylaxis of chronic tension headache. Headache. 1990;30:300.
58. Warner G, Lance JW. Relaxation therapy in migraine and chronic tension headache. Med J Australia. 1975;1:298–301.
59. Daly EJ, Donn PA, Galliher MJ, Zimmerman JS. Biofeedback applications to migraine and tension headache: a double-blinded outcome study. Biofeedback & Self-Regulation 1983;8:135–52.
60. Kaushik R, Kaushik RM, Mahajan SK, Rajesh V. Biofeedback assisted diaphragmatic breathing and systematic relaxation versus propranolol in long term prophylaxis of migraine. Complement Ther Med 2005;13:165–74.
61. Lockett DC, Campbell JF: The effects of aerobic exercise on migraine. Headache 1992;32:50–4.

Chronic Fatigue Syndrome

Key Chapter Points

- Symptoms of extreme, debilitating fatigue are often termed chronic fatigue syndrome in the United States and myalgic encephalitis in the United Kingdom.
- Chronic fatigue syndrome (CFS) affects 2% of adults.
- A combination of both emotional and physical factors likely contributes to the pathogenesis of CFS.
- Graded exercise and cognitive-behavioral therapy effectively reduce fatigue symptoms.
- Antidepressants help reduce non-fatigue, somatic complaints.

Keywords Affective · Anemia · Arthralgia · Immune deficiency · Myalgia

The diagnosis of chronic fatigue has a long and colorful history. Over the years, a variety of terms have been used to describe symptoms of extreme, debilitating fatigue: neurasthenia, neuromyesthenia, and encephalomyelitis. In 1955, a report of an outbreak of an obscure fatigue disorder occurring among staff at the Royal Free Hospital Group in London published in the *British Medical Journal* coined the term Royal Free disease [1].

In the 1980s, chronic fatigue was often attributed to a post-viral fatigue syndrome, especially from chronic Epstein–Barr virus infection after high titers of Epstein–Barr virus antibodies compatible with active infection lasting for at least 1 year were identified in 39 out of 44 patients complaining of chronic fatigue [2]. The term *chronic fatigue syndrome* (CFS) was first used in 1987 [3] and continues to be the favored term in the United States today. The same syndrome is termed *myalgic encephalitis* in the United Kingdom.

Case presentation

Beth is a 57-year-old wife of a family physician with a 5-year history of worsening fatigue, generalized weakness, low-grade subjective fevers, and

D.A. Marcus, A. Deodhar, *Fibromyalgia*, DOI 10.1007/978-1-4419-1609-9_6,
© Springer Science+Business Media, LLC 2011

"enlarged cervical lymph nodes." Her fatigue is "overwhelming, encompassing every aspect of my life!" She had stopping playing golf and volunteering in the local hospital. Her husband reported she snored at night and occasionally woke with choking. A previous extensive work-up, including blood and urine cultures, viral serologies, chest x-rays, an echocardiogram, CT scan of chest, abdomen and pelvis, and lymph node biopsy were all unremarkable and she had been diagnosed with fibromyalgia and CFS. On examination, she was depressed, severely obese (BMI = 35) and had 12 of 18 positive fibromyalgia tender points. A sleep study confirmed sleep apnea, and she was prescribed a CPAP machine. After trying several models, she discontinued CPAP, reporting it made her feel "claustrophobic." In an attempt to treat her sleep apnea, Beth underwent gastric bypass surgery and successfully lost 150 lbs in 16 months. After weight loss, she notice marked improvements in snoring, sleep quality, mood, and fatigue. She reported "feeling like a new woman."

She returned to the clinic 2 years later, still maintaining her new slim figure. She was playing golf three times a week and was active on the managing committee of the golf course. Beth reported a return of fatigue over the previous 4 months, becoming exhausted after playing nine holes of golf. She also complained of "lightheadedness" after being "up on her feet" for several hours. Examination showed a BMI of 26 and blood pressure of 96/60, with only four positive fibromyalgia tender points. A tilt-table test resulted in a drop in systolic blood pressure to 66 mm Hg after vertical positioning for 5 minutes, resulting in a diagnosis of neurally mediated hypotension. She was prescribed compression stockings (10 cm of water pressure) and was asked to increase her daily salt intake. The compression stockings made a dramatic improvement in her energy level. Her fatigue was significantly reduced, she had no more lightheadedness and she was able to enjoy her golf rounds with her friends again. This case illustrates the importance of obtaining a careful history and examination in patients reporting chronic fatigue symptoms to ensure that correctable contributors to fatigue are treated.

Defining Chronic Fatigue Syndrome

The currently accepted standard for defining CFS was established by the International Chronic Fatigue Syndrome Study Group in 1994 (Table 1) [4]. Like fibromyalgia, CFS is more than just a diagnosis of exclusion in patients with fatigue that is unexplained by other medical conditions. It is important to recognize that not all reports of fatigue represent CFS. A survey of 141 patients presenting to their primary care providers with a chief complain of unexplained fatigue lasting at least 6 months found that only 31% of these patients met criteria for a diagnosis of CFS [5]. As illustrated by the case, neurally mediated hypotension, for example,

Table 1 International chronic fatigue syndrome study group CFS definition (based on Fukuda [4])

Required criteria		Exclusionary criteria
Severe, persistent, or relapsing fatigue	*Four or more of the following*:	• Active medical condition that could explain chronic fatigue
• Not lifelong	• Impaired short-term memory or concentration	• Past or current diagnosis of major depressive disorder
• Duration >6 months	• Recurrent sore throat	• Alcohol or substance abuse within 2 years of the onset of CFS
• Not caused by exertion or relieved by rest	• Tender cervical or axillary lymph nodes	• Severe obesity (BMI ≥ 45)
• Associated with disability[a]	• Myalgia	
	• Arthralgia without joint swelling or redness	
	• Headache of new type, pattern, or severity	
	• Non-refreshing sleep	
	• Post-exertional malaise	

[a]Disability defined as substantial reduction in previous levels of occupational, educational, social, and personal activities
BMI = body mass index

often occurs in patients reporting chronic fatigue symptoms, with fatigue frequently improving as autonomic dysfunction is treated [6, 7].

Practical pointer

CFS is characterized by severe, chronic fatigue unrelated to rest and associated with disturbances in cognition, pain, and sleep dysfunction not explained by other active medical conditions.

Patients with CFS typically report other symptoms in addition to fatigue (Box 1). A recent small study comparing memory in 11 women with CFS and 12 controls showed subtle memory decrements in patients with CFS, with significant decreases in free recall. These data help support patient reports of clouded memory [8].

Box 1 Commonly Reported Symptoms in CFS (Based on Hurwitz [26])

- Post-exertional fatigue
- Non-refreshing sleep
- Generalized weakness
- Impaired memory or concentration

- Muscle aches and pain
- Joint pain
- Headaches
- Fevers/chills
- Sore throat
- Tender lymph nodes

Epidemiology of Chronic Fatigue Syndrome

Primary care patients in London ($N = 2,459$) and São Paulo ($N = 3,914$) were surveyed, with CFS identified in 2.1% in Britain and 1.6% in Brazil [9]. Population-based surveys conducted in the United States have likewise reported CFS prevalence of 1.2–2.5% [10, 11].

Practical pointer

CFS affects about 2% of adults.

Fatigue prognosis was evaluated in an observational study of 642 Dutch adults who sought a primary care consultation for a new complaint of fatigue [12]. Fatigue was severe in 90% of patients at the time of the initial consultation. After 1 year, only 45% of those who initially reported severe fatigue were still reporting severe fatigue (Fig. 1). Four patterns of prognosis emerged: continuous severe fatigue in 26%, fast recovery in 17%, slow recovery in 25%, and initial improvement with subsequent recurrence in 32%.

Co-morbidity

Pain and chronic fatigue are frequently co-morbid. In a survey of 2,447 randomly selected adults in a Dutch community sample, persistent fatigue was increasingly common among those with more severe and widespread pain (Fig. 2) [13]. Likewise, chronic, disabling widespread pain was more common among individuals with chronic, disabling fatigue. Chronic fatigue is reported for 81% of patients with fibromyalgia vs. 38% of individuals in the general population [14].

Affective disorders are also co-morbid with CFS. In a survey comparing individuals with CFS and those who were unwell but did not meet criteria for CFS, individuals with CFS were twice as likely to have a psychiatric disorder over their lifetimes and 60% more likely to have a current psychiatric diagnosis [15]. This

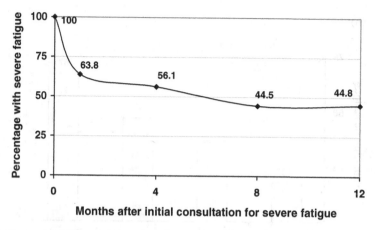

Fig. 1 Prognosis of severe fatigue (based on Nijrolder [12])

increase was due to significantly increased prevalence of both depression and anxiety (Fig. 3). Personality disorders are not more likely to be identified in patients with CFS compared with controls [16].

Practical pointer

Chronic, disabling, widespread pain, depression, and anxiety are co-morbid with CFS.

Pathophysiology of Chronic Fatigue Syndrome

A wide variety of abnormalities have been postulated to result in CFS (Box 2), including both emotional and physical contributing factors [17]. For example, in a study comparing adults with CFS and well controls, adults who had experienced childhood abuse or neglect were twice as likely to have CFS as adults [18]. Conversely, skeletal muscle biopsies from patients with CFS and controls show an increase in the more fatigue-prone, fast fibers, supporting patient complaints of quicker onset fatigue with CFS [19]. It is likely that a combination of factors influence the development of CFS. For example, studies show an increased cumulative allostatic load (physiological effects from the body's adaptive response to exposure to physical and emotional stressors) among individuals with CFS [20].

Genetic factors might also play an important role in CFS, although a family history of CFS is generally lacking. In an interesting recent study, patients with CFS were shown to have a lower expression of beta-2 adrenergic receptors compared with controls at baseline, with similar levels of metabolite and immune genes [21]. After moderate intensity exercise (defined as 70% of maximum age-predicted heart

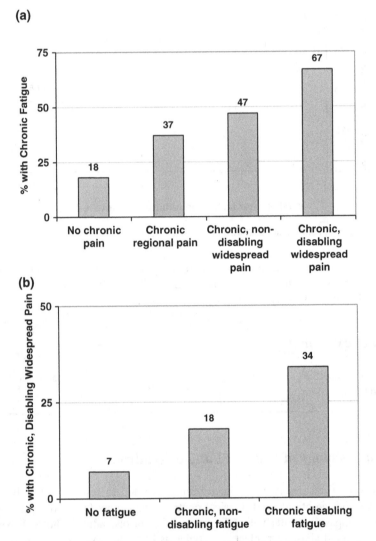

Fig. 2 Chronic fatigue and pain co-morbidity (based on Creavin [13]). (**a**) Prevalence of persistent fatigue based on the presence of pain and (**b**) prevalence of chronic pain based on the presence of persistent fatigue

rate), CFS patients showed enhanced gene expression for receptors detecting muscle metabolites and markers of sympathetic nervous system and immune function (Fig. 4). These changes may suggest a possible mechanism for fatigue after exertion in patients with CFS. Another recent study compared gene expression in blood cells from patients with post-infectious CFS and controls, identifying differentially expressed genes that suggested functional impact for immune modulation, oxidative stress, and apoptosis [22].

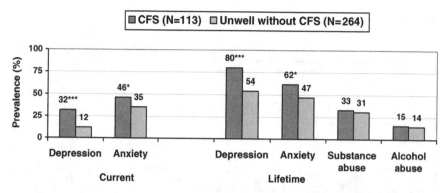

Fig. 3 Psychiatric co-morbidity in CFS compared with unwell persons without CFS (based on Nater [15]). Between-group differences were statistically significant: $*P \leq 0.05$, $***P < 0.001$

Box 2 Proposed Pathophysiology of CFS (Based on Deodhar 2005 [17])

- Post-infection

  - Viral
  - Mycoplasma
  - Chlamydia

- Immune dysfunction
- Chronic non-restorative sleep
- Hypothalamic–pituitary–adrenal axis dysfunction

  - Hypocortisolism
  - Serotonergic dysfunction
  - Growth hormone deficiency

- Dysautonomia
- Psychiatric conditions

  - Mood disorders
  - Anxiety disorders

Role of Immune Deficiency in Chronic Fatigue Syndrome

Although initially linked to infectious immune dysfunction, such as a link to Epstein–Barr infection, the role of possible immune deficiency in CFS remains controversial. In some cases, CFS has been termed *Chronic Fatigue Immune*

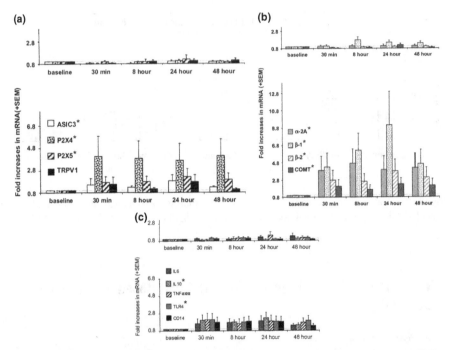

Fig. 4 mRNA at baseline and after moderate exercise in CFS and controls (from Light [21]). In each case, the top figure represents mRNA increases after exercise in the control group, with changes in CFS patients shown in the bottom graph. *$P<0.05$ compared with control subjects for the area under the curve (AUC) of mRNA across all time points after exercise. *Faint dotted line* indicates the baseline levels. ASIC = acid sensing ion channel, P2X = purinergic X type. (**a**) Metabolic detection genes, (**b**) adrenergic function genes, and (**c**) immune function genes

Deficiency Syndrome to highlight the possible role of immune factors. A substantive role of immune factors has gained new strength through research linking xenotropic murine leukemia retrovirus (XMRV) to CFS [23]. Previous work has linked XMRV with prostate cancer [24, 25]. A recent study of peripheral mononuclear cells identified XMRV DNA in 67% of patients with CFS compared with 4% of healthy controls [23]. Furthermore, unaffected blood cells from health controls could become infected after exposure to material from XMRV-positive CFS patients. How the XMRV virus might relate to CFS symptoms is unknown. This virus or other viruses may occur coincidentally, cause direct changes leading to fatigue, or cause indirect changes by inducing transcription of other viruses.

Assessment of Chronic Fatigue Syndrome

There are no diagnostic signs on physical examination and no laboratory tests that can confirm the diagnosis of CFS. All patients reporting symptoms of extreme fatigue should be evaluated with a detailed and thorough history, physical examination, and laboratory tests to rule out significant medical or psychiatric conditions that could explain chronic fatigue symptoms (Box 3).

Box 3 Laboratory Assessment for Chronic Fatigue Symptoms

- Complete blood count
- C-reactive protein
- Blood electrolytes, BUN, and creatinine
- Thyroid functions
- Urinalysis

Anemia may play an important role in the severity of CFS symptoms. In a recently published study, cardiac function was compared in patients with CFS ($N = 56$) and matched healthy controls ($N = 90$) [26]. Echocardiographic measures showed a 10.2% lower cardiac volume and 25.1% lower contractility among those with severe CFS vs. controls. CFS groups also showed lower total blood, plasma, and red blood cell volumes. Analysis suggested that the lower cardiac volumes were a consequence of a co-morbid hypovolemia due to normochromic-normocytic anemia rather than related to diminished cardiac contractility. These data suggest routine screening for anemia should be performed in CFS patients, especially those with more severe symptoms. Viral antibody tests and exhaustive immunological tests are not indicated for the diagnosis of CFS.

Severity of fatigue can be measured using the Fatigue Severity Scale (Table 2) [27]. This scale has been validated in several chronic disease conditions, including CFS, and was recommended for evaluating fatigue severity in CFS by an expert panel [28, 29]. Mean Fatigue Severity Scale Scores were reported in one study as 6.2 ± 0.9 for patients with CFS vs. 3.5 ± 1.4 for patients with sleep apnea vs. 1.7 ± 1.1 for controls [30].

Treatment of Chronic Fatigue Syndrome

Graded exercise and cognitive-behavioral therapy have both shown to be effective in reducing fatigue symptoms and should be offered to patients with CFS (Table 3) [31, 32]. Graded exercise is more effective when patients receive instructions that include training sessions and education about home-based exercise rather than simply written information alone [31].Due to the frequent complaint of post-exertional fatigue in patients with CFS, exercise therapy often needs to vary in intensity, depending on the patient's current symptomatic status. Exercise intensity will differ between patients based on physical capabilities and within the same patient on different days,

Table 2 Fatigue Severity Scale (based on Krupp [27])

	Strongly disagree	Moderately disagree	Mildly disagree	Neither agree nor disagree	Mildly agree	Moderately agree	Strongly agree
	1	2	3	4	5	6	7
My motivation is lower when I am fatigued							
Exercise brings on my fatigue							
I am easily fatigued							
Fatigue interferes with my physical functioning							
Fatigue causes frequent problems for me							
My fatigue prevents sustained physical functioning							
Fatigue interferes with carrying out certain duties and responsibilities							
Fatigue is among my three most disabling symptoms							
Fatigue interferes with my work, family, or social life							

Scoring: add scores for each of the nine questions; divide by 9 for an average Fatigue Severity Scale Score. Higher scores represent higher fatigue

based on symptomatic fluctuations [33]. A suggested scheme for adjusting aerobic activity level based on individual patient abilities is provided in Table 4. Using these restrictions has been shown to successfully prevent important changes in health-related status (as measured by quality of life measures), although an immediate increase in fatigue after exercise is still likely to occur [34].

Practical pointer

Graded exercise is recommended for CFS, although exercise will likely result in short-term increases in fatigue. Exercise success can be maximized by varying exercise intensity based on physical capabilities and symptomatic fluctuations.

Table 3 Efficacy of treatments for CFS (based on Reid [31])

Beneficial	Effectiveness unknown	Not or probably not effective
Cognitive-behavioral therapy Graded exercise	Antidepressants Corticosteroids Dietary supplements Evening primrose Homeopathy Magnesium Nicotinamide adenine dinucleotide Prolonged rest	Galantamine Immunotherapy

Table 4 Suggested scheme for identifying aerobic exercise targets (based on Nijs [33])

Number of minutes able to exercise without flare	Target exercise duration on symptomatically good day	Target exercise duration on symptomatically bad day
Suggested formula # Comfortable minutes	Walk for 75% × (no. of comfortable minutes) Rest for 75% × (no. of comfortable minutes) Walk for 75% × (no. of comfortable minutes)	Walk for 50% × (no. of comfortable minutes) Rest for 50% × (no. of comfortable minutes) Walk for 50% × (no. of comfortable minutes)
Sample patient walking target 20 min	15 min	10 min

The importance of including CBT in a CFS treatment regimen, especially in CFS patients with fibromyalgia, is highlighted by data showing a significant association between pain catastrophizing and bodily pain, exercise performance, and self-reported disability in female patients with CFS and widespread pain [35]. In an interesting study evaluating treatment response in 114 CFS patients, baseline predictors of poor response to psychological treatment included: being a member of a self-help group, receiving sickness benefits, and dysphoria [36]. Patients with co-morbid psychological distress will additionally need therapy targeted to reducing affective symptoms.

While medication effectiveness for fatigue symptoms in CFS has not been established for most drugs (Table 3), medication use is high among patients with chronic fatigue syndrome. In a population-based, case-controlled study, the average number of drugs or supplements used was 5.8 for those with CFS vs. 3.7 for healthy controls [37]. The most frequently used therapies were pain relievers, supplements, allergy medications, antidepressants, and antihistamines (Fig. 5). Despite their limited role in consistently reducing fatigue, antidepressants have been shown to reduce somatic symptoms accompanying CFS [38]. In an interesting 3-year study comparing health status between CFS treated with antidepressants and not treated with antidepressants, patients taking antidepressants at baseline were significantly less likely to report somatic symptoms (e.g., physical weakness, physical fatigue, aching joints, and allergies) at follow-up compared with patients not treated with an antidepressant [39]. Patients treated with an antidepressant were also more likely to report that they were almost recovered at long-term follow-up: 10.5% treated with antidepressants vs. 2.0% without antidepressants at 6 months, 15.8% vs. 6.3% at 18 months, and 29.2% vs. 6.2% at 3 years. A more favorable outcome occurred in those individuals treated with selective serotonin reuptake inhibitors compared with tricyclics. Antidepressants may be a good choice for patients with CFS and fibromyalgia as a recent meta-analysis identified significant improvements in pain, fatigue, sleep disturbance, depression, and quality of life with antidepressant treatment for fibromyalgia [40].

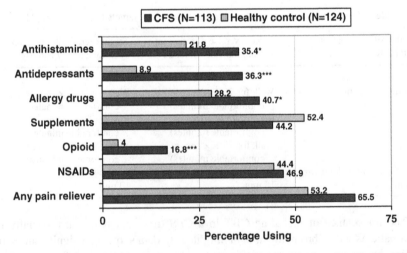

Fig. 5 Medications commonly used by people with CFS vs. controls (based on Boneva [37]). Difference between use in those with CFS and controls was significant: $^*P<0.05$, $^{***}P=0.001$

Summary

- Patients with CFS typically report a variety of symptoms, including fatigue, sleep disturbance, pain, memory or concentration impairments, sore throat, and tender lymph nodes.

- Only one in every three patients seeking medical care for unexplained chronic fatigue will be diagnosed with CFS.
- Chronic fatigue is reported by four of every five patients with fibromyalgia.
- Patients with CFS are 60% more likely to have an ongoing psychiatric condition, especially depression or anxiety.
- Changes in gene expression affecting muscle metabolism, sympathetic nervous system activity, and immune function may influence CFS.
- Antidepressants may reduce somatic symptoms associated with CFS.

References

1. Medical Staff of the Royal Free Hospital. An outbreak of encephalomyelitis in the Royal Free Hospital group, London, in 1955. BMJ. 1957;2:895–904.
2. Jones JF, Ray CG, Minnich LL, Hicks MJ, Kibler R, Lucas DO. Evidence for active Epstein-Barr virus infection in patients with persistent, unexplained illnesses: elevated anti-early antigen antibodies. Ann Intern Med. 1985;102:1–7.
3. Buchwald D, Sullivan JL, Komaroff AL. Frequency of 'chronic active Epstein-Barr virus infection' in a general medical practice. JAMA. 1987;257:2303–7.
4. Fukuda K, Straus SE, Hickie I, Sharpe MC, Dobbins JG, Komaroff A. The chronic fatigue syndrome: a comprehensive approach to its definition and study. International Chronic Fatigue Syndrome Study Group. Ann Intern Med. 1994;121:953–9.
5. Darbishire L, Ridsdale L, Seed PT. Distinguishing patients with chronic fatigue from those with chronic fatigue syndrome: a diagnostic study in UK primary care. Br J Gen Pract. 2003;53:441–5.
6. Rowe PC, Calkins H. Neurally mediated hypotension and chronic fatigue syndrome. Am J Med. 1998;105:15S–21S.
7. Davis Sd, Kator SF, Wonnett JA, Pappas BL, Sall JL. Neurally mediated hypotension in Gulf War veterans: a preliminary report. Am J Med Sci. 2000;319:89–95.
8. Attree EA, Dancey CP, Pope AL. An assessment of prospective memory retrieval in women with chronic fatigue syndrome using a virtual-reality environment: an initial study. Cyberpsychol Behav. 2009;12:379–85.
9. Cho HJ, Menezes PR, Hotopf M, Bhugra D, Wessely S. Comparative epidemiology of chronic fatigue syndrome in Brazilian and British primary care: prevalence and recognition. Br J Psychiatry. 2009;194:117–22.
10. Bierl C, Nisenbaum R, Hoaglin DC, et al. Regional distribution of fatiguing illnesses in the Unites States: a pilot study. Popul Health Metr. 2004;2:1.
11. Reeves WC, Jones JF, Maloney E, et al. Prevalence of chronic fatigue syndrome in metropolitan, urban, and rural Georgia. Popul Health Metr. 2007;5:5
12. Nijrolder I, van der Windt DM, van der Horst HE. Prognosis of fatigue and functioning in primary care: a 1-year follow-up study. Ann Fam Med. 2008;6:519–27.
13. Creavin ST, Dunn KM, Mallen CD, Nijrolder I. Co-occurrence and associations of pain and fatigue in a community sample. Eur J Pain. 2010;14:327–34.
14. Zoppi M, Maresca M. Symptoms accompanying fibromyalgia. Reumatismo. 2008;60:217–20.
15. Nater UM, Lin JM, Maloney EM, et al. Psychiatric comorbidity in persons with chronic fatigue syndrome identified from the Georgia population. Psychosom Med. 2009;71:557–65.
16. Courjaret J, Schotte CK, Wijnants H, Moorkens G, Cosyns P. Chronic fatigue syndrome and DSM-IV personality disorders. J Psychosom Res. 2009;66:13–20.
17. Deodhar A. Chronic Fatigue Syndrome. In: Wallace D, Clauw D, ed. Fibromyalgia and other pain syndromes. Philadelphia: Lippincott Williams & Willkins. 2005;197–208.
18. Heim C, Nater UM, Maloney E, et al. Childhood trauma and risk for chronic fatigue syndrome: association with neuroendocrine dysfunction. Arch Gen Psychiatry. 2009;66:72–80.

19. Pietrangelo T, Tonilol L, Paoli A, et al. Functional characterization of muscle fibres from patients with chronic fatigue syndrome: case-control study. Int J Immunopathol Pharmacol. 2009;22:427–36.

20. Maloney EM, Boneva R, Nater UM, Reeves WC. Chronic fatigue syndrome and high allostatic load: results from a population-based case-control study in Georgia. Psychosom Med. 2009;71:549–56.

21. Light AR, White AT, Hughen RW, Light KC. Moderate exercise increases expression for sensory, adrenergic, and immune genes in chronic fatigue syndrome patients but not in normal subjects. J Pain. 2009;10:1099–1112.

22. Gow JW, Hagan S, Herzyk P, et al. A gene signature for post-infectious chronic fatigue syndrome. BMC Med Genomics. 2009;2:38.

23. Lombardi VC, Ruscetti FW, Das Gupta J, et al. Detection of an infectious retrovirus, XMRV, in blood cells of patients with chronic fatigue syndrome. Science. 2009;326:585–9.

24. Urisman A, Molinaro RJ, Fischer N, et al. Identification of a novel gammaretrovirus in prostate tumors of patients homozygous for R462Q RNASEL variant. PLos Pathog. 2006;2:e25.

25. Dong B, Kim S, Hong S, et al. An infectious retrovirus susceptible to an IFN antiviral pathway from human prostate tumors. Proc Natl Acad Sci USA. 2007;104:1655–60.

26. Hurwitz BE, Coryell VT, Parker M, et al. Chronic fatigue syndrome: illness severity, sedentary lifestyle, blood volume and evidence of diminished cardiac function. Clin Sci (Lond). 2009;118:125–35.

27. Krupp LB et al. The Fatigue Severity Scale: Application to patents with multiple sclerosis and systemic Lupus erythematosus. Arch Neurol. 1989;46:1121–23.

28. Taylor R et al. Fatigue rating scales: an empirical comparison. Psychol Med. 2000;30:849–56.

29. Reeves WC, Lloyd A, Vernon SD, et al. Identification of ambiguities in the 1994 chronic fatigue syndrome research case definition and recommendations for resolution. BMC Health Serv Res. 2003;3:25.

30. Neu D, Hoffmann G, Moutrier R, er al. Are patients with chronic fatigue syndrome just 'tired' or also 'sleepy'? J Sleep Res. 2008;17:427–31.

31. Reid SF, Chalder T, Cleare A, Hotopf M, Wessely S. Chronic fatigue syndrome. Clin Evid BMJ. 2008; pii:1101. (Available at http://online5.hsls.pitt.edu:5828/ceweb/conditions/msd/1101/1101.jsp. Accessed August 2009.)

32. Van Houdenhove B, Luyten P. Customizing treatment of chronic fatigue syndrome and fibromyalgia: the role of perpetuating factors. Psychosomatics. 2008;49:470–77.

33. Nijs J, Paul L, Wallman K. Chronic fatigue syndrome: an approach combining self-management with graded exercise to avoid exacerbations. J Rehabil Med. 2008;40:241–7.

34. Nijs J, Almond F, DeBecker P, Truijen S, Paul L. Can exercise limits prevent post-exertional malaise in chronic fatigue syndrome? An uncontrolled clinical trial. Clin Rehabil. 2008;22:426–35.

35. Nijs J, Van de Putte K, Louckx F, Truijen S, De Meirleir K. Exercise performance and chronic pain in chronic fatigue syndrome: the role of pain catastrophizing. Pain Med. 2008;9:1164–72.

36. Bentall RP, Powell P, Nye FJ, Edwards RT. Predictors of response to treatment for chronic fatigue syndrome. Br J Psychiatry. 2002;181:248–52.

37. Boneva RS, Lin JM, Maloney EM, Jones JF, Reeves WC. Use of medications by people with chronic fatigue syndrome and healthy persons: a population-based study of fatiguing illness in Georgia. Health Qual Life Outcomes. 2009;7:67.

38. Pae CU, Marks DM, Patkar AA, et al. Pharmacological treatment of chronic fatigue syndrome: focusing on the role of antidepressants. Expert Opin Pharmacother. 2009;10:1561–70.

39. Thomas MA, Smith AP. An investigation of the long-term benefits of antidepressant medication in the recovery of patients with chronic fatigue syndrome. Hum Psychopharmacol. 2006;21:503–9.

40. Häuser W, Bernardy K, Üçeyler N, Sommer C. Treatment of fibromyalgia syndrome with antidepressants. A meta-analysis. JAMA. 2009;301:198–209.

Irritable Bowel Syndrome

Key Chapter Points

- Functional gastrointestinal disorders, chronic digestive complaints without identified structural or biochemical pathology, occur in nearly all patients with
fibromyalgia.
- Irritable bowel syndrome and bloating are consistently the most commonly
reported digestive complaints in fibromyalgia patients.
- Two in five patients with fibromyalgia have irritable bowel syndrome (IBS). One
in three patients with IBS has fibromyalgia.
- Patients with suspected IBS will need detailed histories and physical examinations, as well as a battery of basic testing.
- Medication, alternative, and complementary therapies have been shown to help
reduce problematic symptoms in patients with IBS.

Keywords Constipation · Diarrhea · Hypersensitivity · Probiotics

---

Case: Jenny is a 24-year-old graduate student who has complained of intermittent abdominal pain and diarrhea for the last 4 years. "I've had stomach
problems and pain since my junior year in college. The worst pain is in my
hips and it's impossible for me to keep up my weight. My new doctor told me
pain and bowel problems go together in fibromyalgia. So I'm here to get my
fibromyalgia treated."

While intermittent bowel disturbance does occur commonly with
fibromyalgia, doctors need to be vigilant to avoid confusing inflammatory
bowel disease (IBD, like Crohn's disease and ulcerative colitis) associated
with painful enthesitis (inflammation of tendon or ligament insertion sites)
with irritable bowel syndrome and fibromyalgia. Rheumatologists occasionally see patients with spondyloarthritis associated with IBD sent to their
fibromyalgia clinics. These patients typically complain of pain in their "hips."

D.A. Marcus, A. Deodhar, *Fibromyalgia*, DOI 10.1007/978-1-4419-1609-9_7,
© Springer Science+Business Media, LLC 2011

When asked to show where the hip hurts, they characteristically place both their hands on their iliac crests – typical areas of enthesitis. A second clue, also seen in this case, is that IBD patients usually lose weight due to malabsorption, while IBS patients generally gain rather than lose weight.

Gastrointestinal symptoms are among the most common complaints reported in fibromyalgia, with 2 of the top 10 symptoms being digestive complaints: irritable bowel syndrome [IBS] (44% prevalence) and bloating (40% prevalence) [1]. In order to determine if digestive complaints occur in excess with fibromyalgia, the prevalence of functional gastrointestinal disorders was compared in 100 fibromyalgia patients and matched controls [2]. Functional gastrointestinal disorders are chronic digestive complaints that occur without a structural or biochemical cause identified. Patients and controls were 93% female, with an average age of 50 years. Functional gastrointestinal disorders were identified in almost all of the fibromyalgia patients and about one-third of controls (Fig. 1). Individual disorders in each digestive category were additionally significantly more prevalent among fibromyalgia patients. A listing of individual functional gastrointestinal disorders reported by >5% of patients is shown in Table 1. Disorders reported by over one in three patients included incontinence, IBS, and bloating. A variety of other disorders were reported, including some that are described below. Rumination syndrome is characterized by effortless and repeated regurgitation of small amounts of food

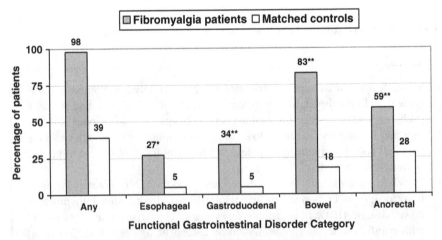

Fig. 1 Prevalence of functional gastrointestinal disorders in fibromyalgia patients vs. matched controls (based on Almansa [2]). Significant differences in prevalence between fibromyalgia patients vs. controls for individual categories: $*P < 0.05$, $**P < 0.001$. Significance for the difference between groups for any disorder was not reported in this study

Table 1 Comparison of individual common (>5% prevalence) functional gastrointestinal disorders between fibromyalgia patients and matched controls (based on Almansa [2])

Functional gastrointestinal disorder	Fibromyalgia (%)	Controls (%)
Esophageal		
Rumination syndrome	8**	0
Dysphagia	6**	0
Gastroduodenal		
Dyspepsia	21**	3
Aerophagia	17**	2
Bowel		
Irritable bowel syndrome	39**	3
Bloating	34**	12
Constipation	15*	5
Anorectal		
Incontinence	45**	25
Levator ani syndrome	23**	4
Proctalgia fugax	10*	1
Pelvic floor dysfunction	7	

Significant differences in prevalence between fibromyalgia patients vs. controls for individual categories: $*P < 0.05$, $**P < 0.001$

from the stomach. The food is then partially or completely rechewed, reswallowed, or expelled. Typically, this occurs without heartburn, abdominal pain, or nausea. Patients with rumination syndrome are often incorrectly diagnosed with gastroesophageal reflux disease or bulimia. Aerophagia occurs when individuals swallow excessive amounts of air into the stomach, resulting in bloating, belching, and pain. Levator ani syndrome describes spasm of the pelvic floor muscles, which causes a fairly constant rectal pressure, tightness, burning, and pain. In contrast, proctalgia fugax (sometimes called anal cramping) is intermittent, severe rectal pain. Episodes often occur at night and last about 15 min. People may say they woke from a sound sleep with a "Charlie horse" or stabbing knife-like pain in their rectum. Pelvic floor dysfunction, also probably related to abnormal muscle spasm, may result in pelvic pain, urinary difficulty, constipation, and pain with intercourse. A subsequent comparative study likewise showed greater severity of belching, reflux, bloating, sour taste, vomiting, and constipation in fibromyalgia patients compared with patients with rheumatoid arthritis or controls ($P<0.01$ for each) [3].

Practical pointer

Digestive complaints are among the most common symptoms in fibromyalgia, most commonly IBS and bloating.

Irritable Bowel Syndrome (IBS)

Definition and Epidemiology

IBS is a common functional bowel disorder characterized by chronic abdominal pain, bloating, and alteration of bowel habits occurring in the absence of gastrointestinal pathology. The diagnosis of IBS has been standardized with the development of the Rome criteria, which were revised in 2006 (Box 1) [4]. Patients may be subclassified into IBS with constipation (IBS-C), with diarrhea (IBS-D), or mixed (IBS-M). IBS-M is comparable to the Rome II category of alternating IBS. General population studies report IBS in 11–20% of adults, with IBS-D the predominant pattern and a female to male ratio of 1.7:1 [5–7]. In an international sample, IBS symptoms occurred an average of 7 days/month with an average of two episodes daily, each lasting approximately 1 h [6].

Box 1 Rome III Criteria for Diagnosis of Irritable Bowel Syndrome

- ≥6 months of abdominal pain
- Abdominal pain fulfilling the following criteria for the last 3 months

  - Symptoms at least 3 days/month
  - At least two of the following:
    - Improvement after defecation
    - Pain onset linked to change in stool frequency
    - Pain onset linked to change in stool appearance

In addition to pain and GI symptoms, individuals with IBS can experience significant disability. In a case-controlled survey, gastrointestinal problems affected daily work performance for 59% with IBS and 17% of controls [8]. Furthermore, short-term sick leave from work due to gastrointestinal problems during the previous year occurred in 24% of individuals with IBS compared with 10% of controls.

IBS is consistently linked with fibromyalgia, occurring in about two of every five fibromyalgia patients [1, 2]. Likewise, among individuals with a primary diagnosis of IBS, one in three also has fibromyalgia [9]. IBS is defined as the combination of recurrent lower abdominal pain and change in bowel habits in patients without identified structural or biochemical pathology.

Practical pointer

Two in five fibromyalgia patients have IBS.
One in three IBS patients has fibromyalgia.

Hypersensitivity to external stimulation reduces pain thresholds for patients with IBS with or without concomitant fibromyalgia [10]. Pain response to both heat and visceral distention was significantly different from controls for both patient groups ($P<0.0001$), with a significant difference for both between patients with IBS alone and IBS plus fibromyalgia ($P\leq0.01$). (See Fig. 2). While hypersensitivity was higher among fibromyalgia patients in both the hand and the feet, patients with IBS alone were more sensitive to visceral distention.

Fig. 2 Pain response to heat and rectal distention (based on Moshiree [10]). Heat stimulation was tested by asking subjects to immerse a hand and then a foot in 45–47°C for 20 s. Visceral distention was performed using a rectal balloon distended for 30 s

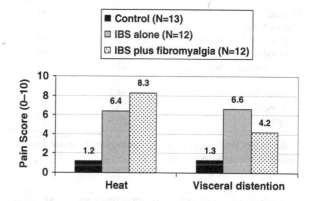

Evaluation and Diagnosis

While abdominal pain is the most common symptom reported by individuals with IBS, a variety of GI symptoms are generally endorsed (Table 2) [6]. Patients reporting symptoms suggestive of IBS will need a detailed history and careful physical examination. Historical features that suggest additional testing may be warranted which include: onset after 50 years old, constitutional symptoms (e.g., unintentional weight loss ≥10 pounds or fever), severe diarrhea, bloody stools, fever, nighttime diarrhea, and a family history of gastrointestinal cancer [11]. Additional testing may also be indicated in patients with an abnormal physical examination. A survey of 806 consecutive patients referred to a specialty gastroenterology practice identified alarm features that suggested organic disease compared with IBS (Table 3) [12].

Table 2 Symptoms commonly reported by individuals with irritable bowel syndrome in a community survey of 41,984 persons in eight European countries (based on Hungin [6])

Symptom	Prevalence (%)
Abdominal pain	88
Bloating	80
Trapped wind	66
Tiredness	60
Diarrhea	59
Tightness of clothing	58
Constipation	53
Heartburn	47

Table 3 Significant predictors of organic lower gastrointestinal disease (based on Hammer [12])

Alarm feature	Prevalence in patients, %		P-value
	IBS	Organic disease	
Age, years			
>45	37.9	56.1	<0.01
>50[a]	23.4	45.5	<0.001
>55	14.5	36.4	<0.001
Female[b]	78.0	51.5	<0.001
Bloody stools			
Blood-coating stools	7.0	19.7	<0.05
Blood mixed with stool	7.9	19.7	<0.01
Blood toilet paper[a]	21.0	42.4	<0.001
Pain			
Severe[b]	54.2	33.3	<0.01
Weekly	74.8	59.1	<0.01
Dysphagia	26.6	13.6	<0.05

[a]Independent predictors of lower gastrointestinal organic disease
[b]Independent predictors of IBS

Table 4 Diagnostic evaluation for patients with symptoms of IBS (based on Olden [11])

Test category	Specific test for patients without alarm features	Additional testing for patients with alarm features
Stool evaluation	Blood Ova and parasites	Not applicable
Laboratory testing	Complete blood count Chemistry panel Erythrocyte sedimentation rate	Thyroid function testing in patients ≥50 years old
Gastrointestinal procedures	Flexible sigmoidoscopy, including biopsy to rule out inflammatory disease or microscopic colitis if diarrhea is present	Colonoscopy in patients ≥50 years old or patients with bloody stools

Independent significant predictors of organic disease were age >50 years old and report of bloody toilet paper, while independent predictors of IBS were female gender and report of severe pain. The presence or absence of alarm features can be used to guide routine testing in patients with symptoms suggesting IBS (Table 4). Screening for thyroid disease and lactose intolerance is best reserved for patients with specific symptoms of these conditions, such as fatigue and weight change (thyroid disease) and intolerance to milk products, including ice cream (lactose intolerance). Patients aged 50 years and older warrant additional screening with a colonoscopy and thyroid function testing. Abdominal ultrasound is generally not helpful.

Practical pointer

Stool and blood analysis plus a sigmoidoscopy are generally considered routine tests in patients reporting symptoms suggesting IBS.

Practical pointer

Additional testing should be considered in patients who are at least 50 years old or reporting unintentional weight loss, bloody stools, fever, nighttime diarrhea, or a family history of colon cancer.

Treatment

Effective IBS treatment will often include a combination of medication, non-medication, and alternative therapies. A variety of effective medications are available, although most treat diarrhea or constipation rather than global IBS symptoms (Table 5) [13–15]. The $5HT_4$ agonist tegaserod [Zelnorm] was withdrawn from the market in the United States and Canada due to an increased risk of cardiovascular

Table 5 Medications for irritable bowel syndrome (IBS) (based on Videlock [13], Holten [14], Spanier [15], Brennan [26])

Medication	Condition improved	Significant side effects
5HT receptor agents		
$5HT_3$ antagonist alosetron [Lotronex]	Global IBS symptoms in women with diarrhea	Constipation
Antidepressants		
Tricyclic	Abdominal pain	Constipation
SSRI	Abdominal pain	Better tolerated than tricyclics
SNRI duloxetine [Cymbalta][a]	Abdominal pain, bloating, and loose stools	Better tolerated than tricyclics
GI		
Loperamide	Diarrhea	Constipation
Fiber/bulking agents	Constipation	Bloating
Oral cromolyn sodium	Diarrhea	Constipation
Selective chloride channel-2 activator lubiprostone [Amitiza]	Constipation	Nausea Diarrhea Headache

5HT = serotonin; SNRI = serotonin norepinephrine reuptake inhibitor; SSRI = selective serotonin reuptake inhibitor
[a]Data from a single, small open-label study treating 14 patients [26]

events. In a recent small study, however, IBS status, FIQ, tender point count, and tender point score were each significantly decreased in fibromyalgia patients treated for 1 month for IBS-C with tegaserod ($P<0.001$ for each) [16]. These data suggest that $5HT_4$ receptor partial agonists may offer benefit to fibromyalgia patients for both digestive complaints and other symptoms of fibromyalgia. Lubiprostone [Amitiza] is approved for the treatment of IBS-C in the United States, with good efficacy with twice daily dosing and improvement persisting for up to 4 weeks after drug discontinuation [17, 18]. Two recent, 12-week, randomized, controlled clinical trials compared efficacy and safety in patients with IBS-C treated with lubiprostone 8 mg or placebo administered twice daily with at least 8 ounces of water at breakfast and dinner ($N = 1,167$) [19]. Most patients were women (92%), with an average age of 47 years. IBS symptoms were moderately or significantly relieved in 18% treated with lubiprostone compared with 10% with placebo ($P = 0.001$). In general, IBS-C symptoms decreased by an average of 1 point on a 5-point severity scale with lubiprostone (representing a clinically meaningful improvement) vs. $\frac{1}{3}$ point with placebo. The most common side effects with lubiprostone were nausea (8% lubiprostone vs. 4% placebo) and diarrhea (6% lubiprostone vs. 4% placebo). Side effects resulted in more discontinuations with placebo (7%) than lubiprostone (5%). Promising emerging therapies for IBS are highlighted in Table 6 [20–24].

A recent meta-analysis of seven double-blind, placebo-controlled trials evaluated the efficacy of tricyclic antidepressants for reducing IBS symptoms [25]. Pooling

Table 6 Emerging therapies for irritable bowel syndrome (based on Lee [20], Andresen [24], Houghton [21], George [23], Gale [22])

Drug category	Specific therapies
5-HT_4 receptor agonists	Prucalopride 2 or 4 mg resulted in normalization of bowel habits in about 20–30% vs. 10% with placebo in clinical trials. Prucalopride 1–2 mg daily (Resolor) has been approved in Europe for the treatment of chronic constipation in women failing to experience adequate relief with laxatives
	TD-5108, ATI-7505, and PF-00885706 are in Phase 2 trials
$5HT_4$ agonist/partial $5HT_3$ antagonist	Renzapride was used to treat IBS-C in a Phase IIb study. Renazpride 4 mg/day resulted in statistically significant improvements in bowel movement frequency and stool consistency
Guanylate cyclase C agonists	Linaclotide 1,000 μg daily for 5 days effectively reduced symptoms in a small sample of 36 women with IBS-C vs. placebo
	Guanilib is in Phase I trials.
Neurostabilizing antiepileptics	Gabapentin (Neurontin) has been shown to reduce visceral hypersensitivity
	Pregabalin (Lyrica) has also been shown to reduce visceral hypersensitivity

data from studies using different tricyclics (amitriptyline, imipramine, desipramine, doxepin, and trimipramine), patients treated with tricyclics were almost twice as likely to experience clinical improvement (relative risk = 1.93; 95% CI 1.4–2.6). Duloxetine was recently tested in a small, 12-week open-label study ($N = 14$; none with co-morbid fibromyalgia) with patients treated with 30 mg daily for 1 week and then 60 mg daily for the remaining 11 weeks. Much to very much improvement was reported by 43% of patients, with significant reductions seen in overall pain (62% decrease, $P<0.001$) and a variety of gastrointestinal symptoms (with decreases of 51% for abdominal pain, 74% for bloating, 71% for loose stool, 62% for urgency, $P<0.01$ for each) [26]. Disability improved 74% for work and family activities ($P<0.01$ for each). While fibromyalgia patients were not included in this small sample, duloxetine may be interesting to consider in fibromyalgia patients with IBS because of its efficacy for also reducing other fibromyalgia symptoms.

Practical pointer

Tegaserod and antidepressants, such as duloxetine, may effectively reduce gastrointestinal and other symptoms in fibromyalgia patients with IBS.

A recent review of published literature provided evidence-based recommendations for inclusion of complementary and alternative treatments in the treatment of IBS (Table 7) [27]. Actual acupuncture has generally shown no additional benefit over a sham acupuncture for IBS. For example, acupuncture failed to show benefit over placebo in a recent study randomizing 230 IBS patients to 3 weeks of treatment

Table 7 Complementary and alternative treatments for irritable bowel syndrome (IBS) (based on Shen [27])

Treatment	Efficacy for IBS
Soluble fiber	Increasing soluble but not insoluble fibers improves constipation and global IBS symptoms. Abdominal pain has not been shown to consistently improve
Peppermint oil	3–6 enteric-coated capsules containing 0.2–0.4 mL peppermint oil daily alleviates IBS and abdominal pain. Capsules need to be swallowed and not chewed to avoid reflux
Herbs	Tong xie yao fang (TXYF), Padma Lax, and STW 5 improve global IBS symptoms
Probiotics	Improves global IBS and abdominal pain. Increase dietary consumption of yogurt, kefir, miso, tempeh, and sauerkraut; supplements also available
Psychological treatments	Strong evidence supports IBS benefits with hypnotherapy. Cognitive-behavioral treatments might also be helpful
Acupuncture	Not beneficial for IBS

with actual acupuncture or sham acupuncture (placebo) [28]. Psychological treatment may be particularly beneficial in IBS treatment as anxiety has been identified in 50% of patients with IBS, with depression in 12% [29]. Including treatment targeted to relieving psychological distress may be especially helpful since GI distress is associated with higher levels of daily stress and psychological distress [30].

> ### Practical pointer
>
> Alternative or complementary treatments with proven efficacy for IBS include soluble fiber, peppermint oil, some herbs, probiotics, and hypnotherapy.

Summary

- 1–2 out of every 10 people surveyed in the general population will have IBS compared with 4 out of 10 fibromyalgia patients.
- One of every three patients with IBS has fibromyalgia.
- Hypersensitivity is increased in patients with IBS, as well as in patients with fibromyalgia.
- Females and patients reporting severe pain are more likely to have IBS than organic disease.
- Most patients with IBS symptoms will need to be evaluated with stool and routine blood testing, as well as a sigmoidoscopy.
- Patients who are at least 50 years old or who report bloody toilet paper will need additional specialized testing. Additional testing may also be warranted in patients with additional medical complaints.
- Among available medication options, tegaserod and antidepressants, such as duloxetine, may effectively reduce gastrointestinal and other, non-digestive fibromyalgia complaints in fibromyalgia patients with IBS.
- Soluble fiber, peppermint oil, some herbs, probiotics, and hyponotherapy are proven non-traditional therapies for IBS. Psychological pain management and treatment directed toward psychological distress may also be beneficial, especially as anxiety and depression occur frequently in patients with IBS.

References

1. Bennett RM, Jones J, Turk DC, Russell IJ, Matallana L. An internet survey of 2,596 people with fibromyalgia. BMC Musculoskeletal Disorders. 2007;8:27.
2. Almansa C, Rey E, Sánchez RG, Sánchez AA, Díaz-Rubio M. Prevalence of functional gastrointestinal disorders in patients with fibromyalgia and the role of psychologic distress. Clin Gastroenterol Hepatol. 2009;7:438–45.

3. Pamuk ON, Umit H, Harmandar O. Increased frequency of gastrointestinal symptoms in patients with fibromyalgia and associated factors: a comparative study. J Rheumatol. 2009;36:1720–4.

4. Rome III. Rome Foundation website: http://www.romecriteria.org/ (Accessed March 2008.)

5. Halder SL, Locke GR, Schleck CD, et al. Natural history of functional gastrointestinal disorders: a 12-year longitudinal population-based study. Gastroenterology. 2007;133:799–807.

6. Hungin AS, Whorwell PJ, Tack J, Mearin F. The prevalence, patterns and impact of irritable bowel syndrome: an international survey of 40,000 subjects. Aliment Pharmacol Ther. 2003;17:643–50.

7. Gómez Alvarez DF, Morales Vargas JG, Rojas Medina LM, et al. Prevalence of irritable bowel syndrome and associated factors according to the Rome III diagnostic criteria in a general population in Colombia. Gatroenterol Hepatol. 2009;32:395–400.

8. Faresjö A, Grodzinsky E, Johansson S, et al. A population-based case-control study of work and psychosocial problems in patients with irritable bowel syndrome – women are more seriously affected than men. Am J Gastroenterol. 2007;102:371–9.

9. Riedl A, Schmidtmann M, Stengel A, et al. Somatic comorbidities of irritable bowel syndrome: a systematic analysis. J Psychosom Res. 2008;64:573–82.

10. Moshiree B, Price DD, Robinson ME, Gaible R, Verne GN. Thermal and visceral hypersensitivity in irritable bowel syndrome patients with and without fibromyalgia. Clin J Pain. 2007;23:323–30.

11. Olden KW. The challenge of diagnosing irritable bowel syndrome. Rev Gastroenterol Dis. 2003;3:S3–11.

12. Hammer J, Eslick GD, Howell SC, Altiparmak E, Talley NJ. Diagnostic yield of alarm features in irritable bowel syndrome and functional dyspepsia. Gut. 2004;53:666–72.

13. Videlock EJ, Chang L. Irritable bowel syndrome: current approach to symptoms, evaluation, and treatment. Gastroenterol Clin N Am. 2007;36:665–85.

14. Holten KB. Irritable bowel syndrome: minimize testing, let symptoms guide treatment. J Fam Pract. 2003;52:942–9.

15. Spanier JA, Howden CW, Jones MP. A systematic review of alternative therapies in the irritable bowel syndrome. Arch Intern Med. 2003;163:265–74.

16. Reitblat T, Zamir D, Polishchuck I, et al. Patients treated by tegaserod for irritable bowel syndrome with constipation showed significant improvement in fibromyalgia symptoms. A pilot study. Clin Rheumatol. 2009;29:1079–82.

17. Owen RT. Lubiprostone – a novel treatment for irritable bowel syndrome with constipation. Drugs Today (Barc). 2008;44:645–52.

18. Lacy BE, Chey WD. Lubiprostone: chronic constipation and irritable bowel syndrome with constipation. Expert Opin Pharmacother. 2009;10:143–52.

19. Drossman DA, Chey WD, Johanson JF, et al. Clinilca trial: lubiprostone in patients with constipation-associated irritable bowel syndrome – results of two randomized, placebo-controlled studies. Alimen Pharmacol Ther. 2009;29:329–41.

20. Lee KJ, Kim JH, Cho SW. Gabapentin reduces rectal mechanosensitivity and increases rectal compliance in patients with diarrhoea-predominant irritable bowel syndrome. Aliment Pharmacol Ther. 2005;22:981–9.

21. Houghton LA, Fell C, Whorwell PJ, et al. Effect of a second-generation alpha2delta ligand (pregabalin) on visceral sensation in hypersensitive patients with irritable bowel syndrome. Gut. 2007;56:1218–25.

22. Gale JD. The use of novel promotility and prosecretory agents for the treatment of chronic idiopathic constipation and irritable bowel syndrome with constipation. Adv Ther. 2009;26:519–30.

23. George AM, Meyers NL, Hickling RI. Clinical trial: renzapride therapy for constipation-predominant irritable bowel syndrome – a multicentre, randomized, placebo-controlled, double-blind study in primary healthcare setting. Aliment Pharmacol Ther. 2008;27: 830–7.

24. Andresen V, Camilleri M, Busciqlio IA, et al. Effect of 5 days linaclotide on transit and bowel function in females with constipation-predominant irritable bowel syndrome. Gastroenterology. 2007;133:761–8.
25. Rahimi R, Nikfar S, Rezaie A, Abdollahi M. Efficacy of tricyclic antidepressants in irritable bowel syndrome: a meta-analysis. World J Gastsroenterol. 2009;15:1548–53.
26. Brennan BP, Fogarty KV, Roberts JL, et al. Duloxetine in the treatment of irritable bowel syndrome: an open-label pilot study. Hum Psychopharmacol. 2009;24:423–8.
27. Shen YA, Nahas R. Complementary and alternative medicine for treatment of irritable bowel syndrome. Can Fam Physician. 2009;55:143–8.
28. Lembo AJ, Conboy L, Kelley JM. A treatment trial of acupuncture in IBS patients. Am J Gastroenterol. 2009;104:1489–97.
29. Mikocka-Walus A, Turnbull D, Moulding N, et al. Psychological comorbidity and complexity of gastrointestinal symptoms in clinically diagnosed irritable bowel syndrome patients. J Gastroenterol Hepatol. 2008;23:1137–43.
30. Hertig VL, Cain KC, Jarrett ME, Burr RL, Heitkemper MM. Daily stress and gastrointestinal symptoms in women with irritable bowel syndrome. Nurs Res. 2007;56:399–406.

Sleep Disturbance

Key Chapter Points

- Sleep disturbance is a frequent co-morbidity in fibromyalgia, with substantial loss of time spent in deeper, restorative stages of sleep.
- Sleep disturbance lowers the pain threshold and deficiencies in deeper, restorative stages of sleep have been linked to the development of musculoskeletal discomfort and mood disturbances typical of fibromyalgia.
- Poor sleep also predicts poorer general health.
- Sleep quality can be reliably measured using an 11-point scale from best (0) to worst possible sleep (10).
- Sleep improves acutely with benzodiazepine receptor agonists or behavioral interventions, although long-term benefits are superior with behavioral interventions.
- Several categories of fibromyalgia treatments, including antidepressants and neuromodulating antiepileptics, result in improvements in both pain and sleep.

Keywords Cardiovascular risk · Diabetes · Insomnia · Obesity · Pain threshold · Sleep assessment

---

Case: Diana is a 47-year-old professional dog groomer and handler whose business showing dogs has been limited by her fibromyalgia symptoms. "I don't know what's worse – the pain or the problems I have sleeping. Every night I lie in bed for hours while my husband snores away. I finally get a couple hours of light sleep before my alarm goes off and when I wake up, I feel more tired than when I went to bed. I think my fibro pain makes it harder to sleep and the worse I sleep the worse my pain gets. It's a vicious cycle. I can't run my business feeling like this! I don't think my pain will get better until I start sleeping, and I'm not going to start sleeping until my pain's better. I guess I'm just doomed!"

D.A. Marcus, A. Deodhar, *Fibromyalgia*, DOI 10.1007/978-1-4419-1609-9_8,
© Springer Science+Business Media, LLC 2011

Sleep needs vary with age, with adults needing to sleep about 7–8 h each night (Box 1). A variety of chemicals that regulate sleep (e.g., cortisol, growth hormone, and melatonin) vary with age, causing significant changes in sleep patterns with aging [1–4]. Typical sleep in adults occurs in cycles involving sequential sleep phases (Table 1). Non-REM sleep generally lasts for about 90 min before REM sleep occurs. Sleepwalking can occur during the deep sleep that occurs before REM sleep. During REM sleep, voluntary muscles are paralyzed; experts postulate that lack of movement during dream sleep prevents sleepers from harming themselves while acting out dreams. Adults spend about 75–80% of their sleep time in non-REM sleep and 20–25% in REM sleep. With aging, sleep stages 3 and 4 shorten dramatically, shifting seniors toward lighter, less restful stages of sleep.

Box 1 Nightly Sleep Requirements at Different Ages

- Newborns – 16–20 h
- Toddler – 10–12 h
- Elementary student – 10 h
- Teenager – more than 9 h
- Adult – 7–8 h

Table 1 Normal sleep stages

Sleep stage	Features
Non-REM 75–80% of sleep time for normal adults	
1	Light sleep. May experience feeling of falling and involuntarily jerk and waken. Eyes are closed, but if woken during this stage, people often feel like they have not slept
2	Light sleep. Heart rate slows and body temperature decreases in preparation for deeper stages of sleep
3	Deeper sleep. May feel temporarily confused and disoriented for a few minutes if wake during this stage
4	Deeper sleep. May feel temporarily confused and disoriented for a few minutes if wake during this stage
REM 20–25% of sleep time for normal adults	Increased breathing and heart rate. No extremity movement. Dreams occur

REM = rapid eye movement

Sleep disturbance may involve problems with sleep quantity or quality. Insomnia may be diagnosed in patients with insufficient sleep quantity (with difficulty initiating and/or maintaining sleep) or sleep quality (experiencing restless or light sleep, called non-restorative sleep). In both cases, sleep impairment is associated with daytime impairment or distress. The National Sleep Foundation surveys adults in the United States using the Sleep in America poll to determine sleep quantity and impact from sleep deficiencies [5]. In the most recent survey, the average American slept 6 h and 40 min at night on weekdays and 7 h and 25 min at night on the weekends. Interestingly, these same people reported needing to sleep 7 h and 18 min on average to function at their best. Sequential surveys by the National Sleep Foundation clearly document that poor sleep is increasing. In 1998, one in every three adults reported sleeping 8 or more hours per night on week nights, dropping to only one in four adults in 2005. In the 2008 survey, poor sleep was linked to difficulties with daily tasks with poor sleep resulting in work tardiness during the preceding month for 1 in 10 adults and falling asleep or being very sleepy on the job for almost one in three adults. Sleep quality was assessed in a large survey of 25,580 Europeans from seven countries, with non-restorative sleep in 11% of people [6]. Those with non-restorative sleep were over twice as likely to report moderate-to-severe physical and intellectual fatigue and over three times more likely to report a moderate-to-severe decrease in effectiveness, memory problems, and mood problems (including irritability, depression, and anxiety).

Consequences of Sleep Disturbance

In one study, students (ages 17–30 years) sleeping only 6–7 h nightly were 50% more likely to report having poor health compared with those getting a full night's sleep [7]. Individuals sleeping <6 h nightly were twice as likely to have poor health. Similarly, a large survey of over 200 million adults in the United States found that almost one in five had trouble sleeping [8]. Those individuals with sleep problems were more likely to have obesity, high blood pressure, congestive heart failure, anxiety, and depression.

Sleep affects a variety of physiological systems in the body:

- Appetite suppression [9]
- Blood glucose regulation [10]
- Catecholamines [11]
- Immune-mediating hormones (e.g., corticotrophin-releasing hormone, growth hormone, cortisol, and prolactin) [12, 13]
- Pain threshold [14]

Possibly because of the wide-reaching physiological effects of sleep, sleep disturbance has been linked to a myriad of health risks, including cardiovascular disease, obesity, diabetes, and pain. For example, sleep disturbance causes an increase in inflammatory markers, including interleukin-1 and interleukin-6 [15]. Increases in proinflammatory cytokines that occur with sleep deprivation have been linked to increased risk for arthritis, cardiovascular disease, and diabetes [16]. Interestingly, women are more sensitive to this inflammatory response with sleep disturbance, suggesting that sleep regulation may be even more important in women to avoid health risks from poor sleep [17].

Cardiovascular Disease

Sleep disturbance has been linked to cardiovascular disease in large population samples. For example, people typically sleeping 5 or fewer hours per night were over twice as likely to have high blood pressure compared with people sleeping 7–8 h per night in a study of 3,620 adults between ages 32 and 59 years old [18]. Long-term effects of sleep deprivation on the heart were studied in a group of over 70,000 nurses followed for 10 years [19]. Those women sleeping 5 or fewer hours each night had almost twice the risk of experiencing heart disease compared with women sleeping 8 h at night. Sleep loss also increases chemicals that cause inflammation, which is another important risk factor for heart disease, as well as arthritis and diabetes [20].

> **Practical pointer**
>
> Poor sleep results in increased levels of harmful inflammatory markers and increased risk for hypertension and heart disease.

Obesity

Researchers at Columbia University monitored weight over 10 years in adults in the United States [21]. People who reported sleeping less than 7 h per night were more likely to develop obesity compared with people who slept 7 or more hours nightly. The less people slept, the more overweight they were. Excess weight was highest in those people sleeping the fewest hours each night. People sleeping only 2–4 h each night were over twice as likely to be obese as people sleeping 7 h or more. The risk for being obese was 60% higher in people sleeping 5 h each night and 27% higher among those sleeping 6 h.

> **Practical pointer**
>
> Sleep acts as an appetite suppressant and sleep deprivation increases the risk for obesity.

Diabetes

Longitudinal effects of sleep patterns on risk for diabetes were evaluated in a survey of about 1,200 adults who were re-assessed after 12 years [22]. Men sleeping ≤5 h nightly had a nearly three times greater risk of developing diabetes. Furthermore, men reporting difficulty staying asleep were almost five times more likely to develop diabetes. Interestingly, women with sleep problems did not have a higher risk for developing diabetes. A similar study of over 1,500 men followed for about 16 years in the United States likewise found that men sleeping ≤6 h nightly were twice as likely to develop diabetes [23]. In their survey, those men with excessive sleep (>8 h nightly) also had a higher risk of developing diabetes. In addition, sleep deprivation has been linked to poorer blood sugar control among individuals with diabetes [24]. Furthermore, diabetics with a higher sleep debt are more likely to have major diabetes complications of the peripheral nerves, retina, kidneys, or heart.

Practical pointer

Sleep affects blood glucose, with risk for developing diabetes doubled in men sleeping ≤6 hours per night and tripled in men sleeping ≤5 hours per night. Diabetes risk has not been linked to sleep for women.

Pain Sensitivity

Sleep deficiencies have been linked to a reduced pain threshold. Pain threshold was measured in healthy adults assigned to different sleep conditions [25]. Pain threshold was lowered by one-fourth among people allowed to spend only 4 h in bed at night compared with those allowed to spend 8 h in bed. Furthermore, pain threshold was decreased by one-third in individuals who experienced disrupted sleep with lack of normal non-REM–REM cycling. These experiments show that either reduced sleep quantity or poor quality increased pain sensitivity.

Practical pointer

Insufficient sleep quantity or quality is linked to increased pain sensitivity.

Sleep Disturbance in Fibromyalgia

Sleep disturbance is frequently co-morbid with chronic pain conditions. In a recent review, the prevalence of chronic insomnia was over three times greater among those with chronic pain compared with those without a pain condition (50% vs. 18%, P<0.001) [26]. Fibromyalgia patients likewise frequently report co-morbid sleep dysfunction. In one study of 67 fibromyalgia patients (97% female, mean age 56 years), sleep disturbance was noted for 81% vs. 32% of people in the general population [27]. Similar significant impairments in sleep were identified in a comparison between two large fibromyalgia cohorts enrolled in clinical trials and a general population sample using the validated Medical Outcomes Study Sleep Scale (Fig. 1) [28].

Practical pointer

Poor sleep affects four of every five patients with fibromyalgia.

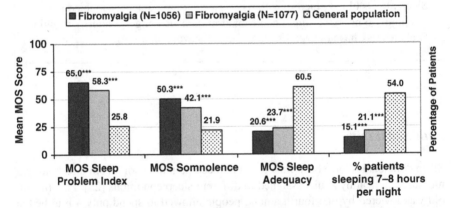

Fig. 1 Sleep disturbance in fibromyalgia patients in two clinical trials and a general population sample (based on Cappelleri [28]). Mean scores based on Medical Outcomes Study Sleep Scale. Higher values for MOS Sleep Problem Index and Somnolence represent a greater sleep disturbance. Lower scores on MOS Sleep Adequacy represent a greater sleep disturbance. All differences between fibromyalgia patients and the general population were significant (***P<0.001)

Loss of restorative, deep sleep has long been linked to fibromyalgia. Sleep studies were compared in patients with fibromyalgia and healthy controls [29]. Sleep recorded for fibromyalgia patients revealed a paucity of time spent in stages 3 and 4 of sleep compared with baseline sleep among the healthy controls (Fig. 2). Among healthy controls, about 4 h were spent in lighter stages of non-REM sleep (stages 1 and 2), 1.5 h in deep, restorative sleep (stages 3 and 4), and 1.5 h in REM sleep. Fibromyalgia patients spent an average of 3.5 h in light non-REM stages 1 and 2,

Fig. 2 Sleep architecture in
fibromyalgia patients
compared with healthy
controls (based on Moldofsky
[29]). (a) Healthy controls:
total sleep time = 435 min,
(b) fibromyalgia patients:
total sleep time = 368 min

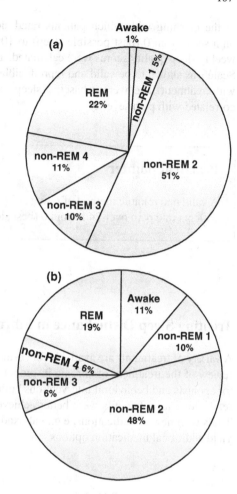

45 min in restorative stages 3 and 4, and 1 h in REM sleep. Following stage 4 deprivation in healthy controls, healthy controls developed musculoskeletal discomfort and mood disturbance, similar to that seen in the fibromyalgia patients, suggesting an important causative or aggravating role for sleep disturbance in fibromyalgia. Deficiencies in non-restorative sleep (during which growth hormone is released) may also explain the link between growth hormone deficiency and fibromyalgia described in the chapter "Pathophysiology of Fibromyalgia".

Measuring Sleep Dysfunction in Fibromyalgia Patients

Sleep was assessed in fibromyalgia patients participating in two randomized, controlled clinic trials, using a single-item Sleep Quality Scale completed on rising in the morning with which patients rated sleep quality over the preceding 24 h on a scale from 0 (best possible sleep) to 10 (worst possible sleep) [30]. Average weekly sleep quality scores were calculated. The single answer to the Sleep Quality Scale was shown to be valid and reproducible and also responsive to sleep changes with treatment. The average baseline sleep score was 7. Furthermore, sleep quality correlated with pain severity.

Practical pointer

A valid and reliable method of rating sleep is through the Sleep Quality Scale. Patients rate pain over 24 h from 0 (best sleep) to 10 (worst sleep).

Treating Sleep Disturbance in Fibromyalgia

A variety of treatments are available for co-morbid insomnia (Table 2) [31]. A recent review of the treatment of chronic insomnia concluded that benzodiazepine receptor agonists and behavioral interventions both offered effective short-term insomnia relief; long-term benefits were better achieved with behavioral interventions [32]. Trials with newer medications, e.g., gaboxadol, tasimelteon, and agomelatine, may yield additional medication options.

Table 2 Treatments for co-morbid insomnia

Treatment category	Individual options
Medications FDA-approved for insomnia	
Benzodiazepine receptor agonists	
Benzodiazepine	Estazolam, flurazepam, quazepam, temazepam, triazolam
Nonbenzodiazepines	Eszopiclone, zaleplon, zolpidem
Melatonin receptor agonist	Ramelteon
Medications with beneficial sedating side effects	
Antidepressants	Tricyclics, trazodone
Neuromodulating antiepileptics	Gabapentin, pregabalin
Muscle relaxants	Tizanidine
Non-medication behavioral interventions	
Sleep hygiene	Sleep scheduling, stimulus control
Relaxation techniques	Progressive muscle relaxation, deep breathing, biofeedback

Medication

While insomnia-specific therapies (e.g., benzodiazepine receptor agonists) may provide good short-term relief of sleep disturbance, medications selected for long-term treatment of insomnia would ideally favor those that can effectively reduce other fibromyalgia symptoms in addition to insomnia. Antidepressants (including tricyclics, selective serotonin reuptake inhibitors, and dual serotonin and noradrenaline reuptake inhibitors) have a strong track record for sleep improvement in patients with fibromyalgia [33]. Likewise, neuromodulating antiepileptics gabapentin and pregabalin have been shown in randomized controlled trials to significantly reduce both pain and sleep disturbance in fibromyalgia patients [34]. In a recent study, pregabalin was shown to significantly improve sleep, especially at total daily doses of 450 and 600 mg; with this effect independent of pregabalin's analgesic properties [35]. Although not specifically tested in fibromyalgia patients, the muscle relaxant tizanidine has been shown to reduce both pain and sleep disturbance in patients with myofascial pain [36]. Tizanidine, therefore, may be considered in fibromyalgia patients with co-morbid myofascial pain and insomnia who have failed to achieve benefit from antidepressants or antiepileptics.

The importance of sleep in fibromyalgia has been highlighted in data showing that treatment with the narcolepsy drug sodium oxybate (Xyrem®) effectively reduces sleep abnormalities, fatigue, and pain in patients with fibromyalgia [37, 38]. A recently published, large, randomized, double-blind, placebo-controlled trial ($N = 188$) reported benefit with 4.5 or 6 g sodium oxybate nightly for 8 weeks (Fig. 3) [35]. Sodium oxybate was generally well tolerated, with discontinuations due to adverse events occurring for 5% with placebo, 9% with sodium oxybate 4.5 g, and 18% with sodium oxybate 6 g.

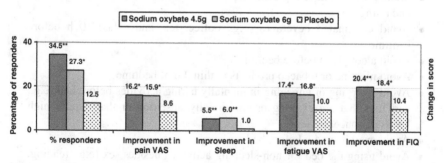

Fig. 3 Treatment outcome with sodium oxybate vs. placebo (based on Russell [35]). Response was defined using a composite of improvement in pain, disability, and global impression. Pain and fatigue were rated using Visual Analogue Scales from 0 to 100. Sleep was scored using the Jenkins Scale for Sleep (ranging from 0 to 20). Disability was rated using the fibromyalgia impact questionnaire (FIQ; range 0–100). Changes in score were significantly different from changes with placebo: *$P \leq 0.05$, **$P < 0.01$

Behavioral Inventions

Instruction in behavioral interventions may be delivered by trained nurses, psychologists, or other therapists. Recently, a randomized controlled trial demonstrated benefit from participation in an online treatment that included sleep education, sleep hygiene instruction, cognitive therapy, relaxation training, and medication tapering [39].

Sleep Hygiene Measures

A variety of sleeping habits have been linked to better sleep quality (Box 2) [40]. In an interesting comparison between individuals with good and poor sleep, analyses of each of these behaviors revealed that those with poor sleep were significantly more likely to [40]:

- Nap during the day
- Engage in activating or arousing activities before bed
- Worry, plan, or think about important matters at bedtime
- Use bed for non-sleep activities (e.g., reading, watching television, or lounging)
- Have an uncomfortable bed environment (e.g., uncomfortable mattress, excessive noise or lighting, or uncomfortable temperature)

Box 2 Good Sleep Hygiene Practices (Based on Gellis [40])

- Avoid excessive daytime napping
- Maintain a regular sleep schedule with consistent times for going to bed and rising
- Avoid caffeinated beverages (e.g., coffee, tea, and colas) 10 h before bedtime
- Avoid alcohol 3 h before bedtime
- Avoid nicotine or tobacco products within 2 h of bedtime
- Avoid worrying or engaging in mentally taxing activities before bed (e.g., activities that are exciting or emotionally upsetting or that require high levels of concentration)
- Avoid exercising 4 h before bed
- Avoid using the bed for non-sleeping activities besides sex (e.g., reading, watching television, lounging)
- Use a comfortable mattress
- Adjust room lighting and noise so that it is conducive to sleep
- Avoid uncomfortable nighttime temperatures

While this study did not directly examine the effects of sleep of changing these behaviors, most experts agree that adopting healthier sleep habits generally improves sleep quality.

Bedtime should be scheduled and associated with a calming routine. Practicing gentle stretching and deep breathing or relaxation exercises before bed can help prepare the body and mind for sleep. Dimming lighting and lowering volumes of radios and televisions about 1 h before the scheduled bedtime can also assist. Patients can also be encouraged to place their lights on a timer to begin to turn on about 30–60 min before rise time in the morning to help prepare the brain for waking up before the alarm blares.

Cognitive-Behavioral Therapy

Cognitive-behavioral therapy includes specific instruction to change a patient's thoughts about a health problem. Adding cognitive therapy to sleep hygiene instruction results in significantly better sleep improvement compared with sleep hygiene education alone [41]. In an interesting controlled study, cognitive-behavioral therapy alone ($N = 80$) or in conjunction with the benzodiazepine receptor agonist zolpidem 10 mg daily ($N = 80$) were tested for short-term and long-term sleep impact [42]. The cognitive-behavioral component was administered by a trained psychologist and included instruction in sleep hygiene and therapy to correct sleep misconceptions (e.g., unrealistic sleep expectations and catastrophizing about sleep disturbance). Patients in both treatment groups experienced significant improvements in sleep. Overall, insomnia improved substantially in 60% of patients after 6 weeks and 65% after 6 months, with insomnia remission achieved by 42% after 6 weeks and 51% after 6 months. Adding zolpidem provided modest additional improvements at 6 weeks (especially with increased sleep time), although better long-term outcomes were achieved when zolpidem was discontinued after the initial 6-week trial.

Practical pointer

Adding benzodiazepine receptor agonists to behavioral interventions produces modest added short-term improvement in sleep disturbance, although long-term benefit is better in patients relying on behavioral intervention.

Natural Remedies

Small, open-label studies treating fibromyalgia patients with melatonin 3–6 mg nightly have reported improvements in sleep, as well as reductions in pain and tender point counts and scores [43]. Trials specifically testing melatonin agonist ramelteon are not yet available, although this treatment may also be helpful.

Acupuncture has been studied in a number of trials, with positive benefits reported; a recent review of these trials, however, concluded that the significant methodological flaws of the studies prevented concluding that acupuncture is beneficial for insomnia until well-controlled, blinded trials support the results of currently available studies [44].

Summary

- Sleep disturbance is reported by 80% of fibromyalgia patients.
- Sleep disturbance has been linked to increased risk of a variety of health problems, including cardiovascular disease, obesity, and diabetes. Sleep disturbance also lowers the pain threshold.
- The Sleep Quality Scale is a valid and reproducible measure of sleep, asking patients to rate sleep quality over the preceding 24 h from 0 (best possible sleep) to 10 (worst possible sleep).
- Benzodiazepine receptor agonists offer short-term sleep improvement.
- Long-term benefit may be achieved with behavioral interventions and some fibromyalgia medications (e.g., antidepressants or antiepileptics). Sleep benefits with pregabalin have been shown to be independent of pain relief.
- Nighttime dosing with melatonin has shown promise in small, open-label studies for reducing both sleep disturbance and pain.

References

1. Prinz PN, Bailey SL, Woods DL. Sleep impairments in healthy seniors: roles of stress, cortisol, and interleukin-1 beta. Chronobiol Int. 2000;17:391–404.
2. Blackman MR. Age-related alterations in sleep quality and neuroendocrine function. Interrelationships and implications. JAMA. 2000;284:879–81.
3. Cajochen C, Münch M, Knoblauch V, Blatter K, Wirz-Justice A. Age-related changes in the circadian and homestatic regulation of human sleep. Chronobiol Int. 2006;23:461–74.
4. Van Cauter E, Leproult R, Plat L. Age-related changes in slow wave sleep and REM sleep and relationship with growth hormone and cortisol levels in healthy men. JAMA. 2000;284: 861–8.
5. National Sleep Foundation 2008 Sleep in America Poll. Available at www.sleepfoundation.org. Accessed July 2008.
6. Ohayon MM. Prevalence and correlates of nonrestorative sleep complaints. Arch Intern Med. 2005;165:35–41.
7. Steptoe A, Peacey V, Wardle J. Sleep duration and health in young adults. Arch Intern Med. 2006;166:1689–92.
8. Pearson NJ, Johnson LL, Nahin RL. Insomnia, trouble sleeping, and complementary and alternative medicine. Analysis of the 2002 National Health Interview Survey. Arch Int Med. 2006;166:1775–82.
9. Vanitallie TB. Sleep and energy balance: interactive homeostatic systems. Metabolism. 2006;55:S30–5.

10. Spiegel K, Knutson K, Leproult R, Tasali E, Van Cauter E. Sleep loss: a novel risk factor for insulin resistance and Type 2 diabetes. J Appl Physiol. 2005;99:2008–19.

11. Takase B, Akima T, Satomura K, et al. Effects of chronic sleep deprivation on autonomic activity by examining heart rate variability, plasma catecholamine, and intracellular magnesium levels. Biomed Pharmacother. 2004;58:S35–9.

12. Bryant PA, Trinder J, Curtis N. Sick and tired: does sleep have a vital role in the immune system? Nat Rev. 2004;4:457–67.

13. Lange T, Dimitriov S, Fehm H, Westermann J, Born J. Shift of monocyte function toward cellular immunity during sleep. Arch Intern Med. 2006;116:1695–700.

14. Roehrs T, Hyde M, Blaisdell B, Greenwald M, Roth T. Sleep loss and REM sleep loss are hyperalgesic. Sleep. 2006;29:145–51.

15. Prather AA, Marsland AL, Hall M, et al. Normative variation in self-reported sleep quality and sleep debt is associated with stimulated pro-inflammatory cytokine production. Biol Psychol. 2009;82:12–17.

16. Mullington JM, Haack M, Toth M, Serrador JM, Meier-Ewert HK. Cardiovascular, inflammatory, and metabolic consequences of sleep deprivation. Prog Cardiovasc Dis. 2009;51: 294–302.

17. Irwin MR, Carrillo C, Olmstead R. Sleep loss activates cellular markers of inflammation: sex difference. Brain Behav Immun. 2010;24:54–7.

18. Gangwisch JE, Heymsfield SB, Boden-Albala B, et al. Short sleep duration as a risk factor for hypertension. Analyses of the first National Health and Nutrition Examination Survey. Hypertension. 2006;47:833–9.

19. Ayas NT, White DP, Manson JE, et al. A prospective study of sleep duration and coronary heart disease in women. Arch Intern Med. 2003;163:205–9.

20. Irwin MR, Wang M, Campomayor CO, Collado-Hidalgo A, Cole S. Sleep deprivation and activation of morning levels of cellular and genomic markers of inflammation. Arch Intern Med. 2006;166:1756–62.

21. Gangwisch JE, Malaspina D, Boden-Albala B, Heymsfield SB. Inadequate sleep as a risk factor for obesity: analyses of the NHANES I. Sleep. 2005;28:1289–96.

22. Mallon L, Broman J, Hetta J. High incidence of diabetes in men with sleep complaints or short sleep duration. Diabetes Care. 2005;28:2762–7.

23. Yaggi HK, Araujo AB, McKinlay JB. Sleep duration as a risk factor for the development of Type 2 diabetes. Diabetes Care. 2006;29:657–61.

24. Knutson KL, Ryden AM, Mander BA, van Cauter E. Role of sleep duration and quality in the risk and severity of Type 2 diabetes mellitus. Arch Intern Med. 2006;166: 1768–74.

25. Roehrs T, Hyde M, Blaisdell B, Greenwald M, Roth T. Sleep loss and REM sleep loss are hyperalgesic. Sleep. 2006;29:145–51.

26. Roth T. Comorbid insomnia: current directions and future challenges. Am J Manag Care. 2009;15:S6–13.

27. Zoppi M, Maresca M. Symptoms accompanying fibromyalgia. Reumatismo. 2008;60: 217–20.

28. Cappelleri JC, Bushmakin AG, McDermott AM, et al. Measurement properties of the Medical Outcomes Study Sleep Scale in patients with fibromyalgia. Sleep Med. 2009;10: 766–70.

29. Moldofsky H, Scarisbrick P, England R, Smythe H. Musculoskeletal symptoms and non-REM sleep disturbance in patients with "fibrositis syndrome" and healthy subjects. Psychosom Med. 1975;37:341–51.

30. Cappelleri JC, Bushmakin AG, McDermott AM, et al. Psychometric properties of a single-item scale to assess sleep quality among individuals with fibromyalgia. Health Qual Life Outcomes. 2009;7:54.

31. Neubauer DN. Current and new thinking in the management of comorbid insomnia. Am J Manag Care. 2009;15:S24–32.

32. Riemann D, Perlis ML. The treatments of chronic insomnia: a review of benzodiazepine receptor agonists and psychological and behavioral therapies. Sleep Med Rev. 2009;13: 205–14.

33. Uçeyler N, Häuser W, Sommer C. A systematic review on the effectiveness of treatment with antidepressants in fibromyalgia syndrome. Arthritis Care Res. 2008;59:1279–98.

34. Häuser W, Bernardy K, Uçeyler N, Sommer C. Treatment of fibromyalgia syndrome with gabapentin and pregabalin – A meta-analysis of randomized controlled trials. Pain. 2009;145:69–81.

35. Russell IJ, Crofford LJ, Leon T, et al. The effects of pregabalin on sleep disturbance symptoms among individuals with fibromyalgia syndrome. Sleep Med. 2009;10:604–10.

36. Malanga GA, Gwynn MW, Smith R, Miller D. Tizanidine is effective in the treatment of myofascial pain syndrome. Pain Physician. 2002;5:422–32.

37. Scharf MB, Baumann M, Berkowitz DV. The effects of sodium oxybate on clinical symptoms and sleep patterns in patients with fibromyalgia. J Rheumatol. 2003;30:1070–4.

38. Russell IJ, Perkins AT, Michalek JE. Sodium oxybate relieves pain and improves function in fibromyalgia syndrome: a randomized, double-blind, placebo-controlled, multicenter clinical trial. Arthritis Rheum. 2009;60:299–309.

39. Vincent N, Lewycky S. Logging on for better sleep: RCT fo the effectiveness of online treatment for insomnia. Sleep. 2009;32:807–15.

40. Gellis LA, Lichstein KL. Sleep hygiene practices of good and poor sleepers in the United States: an Internet-based study. Behav Ther. 2009;40:1–9.

41. Edinger JD, Olsen MK, Stechuchak KM, et al. Cognitive behavioral therapy for patients with primary insomnia or insomnia associated predominantly with mixed psychiatric disorders: a randomized clinical trial. Sleep. 2009;32:499–510.

42. Morin CM, Vallières A, Guay B, et al. Cognitive behavioral therapy, singly and combined with medication, for persistent insomnia: a randomized controlled trial. JAMA. 2009;301:2005–15.

43. Reiter RJ, Acuna-Castroviejo D, Tan DX. Meatlonin therapy in fibromyalgia. Curr Pain Headache Rep. 2007;11:339–42.

44. Yeung WF. Chung KF. Leung YK, Zhang SP. Law AC. Traditional needle acupuncture treatment for insomnia: a systematic review of randomized controlled trials. Sleep Med. 2009;10:694–704.

Depression and Anxiety

Key Chapter Points

- Treatment-seeking patients with fibromyalgia have significantly more psychiatric co-morbidity compared with fibromyalgia non-patients or healthy controls.
- Fibromyalgia patients should be routinely screened for psychological distress.
- Disruptive mood disorders will need to be directly treated in addition to other fibromyalgia treatments.
- Both medication and non-medication fibromyalgia treatments have been shown to improve symptoms of pain and psychological distress.

Keywords Locus of control · Mood disorder · Personality disorder · Self-efficacy

Case: Anna Mae is a 34-year-old accountant and mother of three who was diagnosed with fibromyalgia after her second child was born 7 years ago. She becomes teary-eyed when telling the doctor how fibromyalgia symptoms caused her to miss her son's soccer game. When asked how her mood has been, she sobs, "Everybody just thinks it's all in my head and I'm just depressed! I'm not depressed – I'm having pain! If you'd just get rid of my fibromyalgia, my mood would be fine." Further questioning reveals that she has been having frequent episodes of crying, difficulty sleeping, and has unintentionally lost 15 pounds, which she attributes to loss of appetite and interest in food. Anna Mae also quit volunteering with her daughter's dance group "because I just wasn't interested in doing it anymore." She has also dropped out of an evening exercise program and usually retreats to her bedroom as soon as the family has been fed.

This case illustrates the frequent co-occurrence of fibromyalgia and mood disturbance, both of which can add substantially to the misery and disability of this chronic pain disorder. While patients may feel that mood disturbance has occurred as a reaction to their fibromyalgia symptoms, it is important to

D.A. Marcus, A. Deodhar, *Fibromyalgia*, DOI 10.1007/978-1-4419-1609-9_9,
© Springer Science+Business Media, LLC 2011

additionally identify and address psychological distress as these symptoms are often treatable and failure to treat will likely delay improvement in other fibromyalgia symptoms.

Epidemiology

Psychiatric co-morbidity is common in patients with fibromyalgia. A study of 30 consecutive outpatients with fibromyalgia revealed frequent co-morbidity with depression, anxiety, and personality disorders (Fig. 1) [1]. Despite these links, fibromyalgia should not itself be considered to be primarily a psychological or psychiatric disorder. Indeed, psychiatric co-morbidity reflects greater symptom severity identified in treatment seekers, without a strong link identified with fibromyalgia when considering community samples.

Practical pointer

Depression or anxiety affects almost two in every three patients with fibromyalgia.

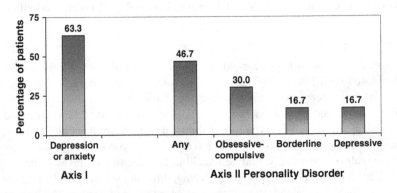

Fig. 1 Psychiatric co-morbidity with fibromyalgia (based on Rose [1])

When linking psychiatric co-morbidity with fibromyalgia, it is important to recognize that symptoms in fibromyalgia treatment seekers do not necessarily reflect symptoms reported by individuals with fibromyalgia in the community. Treatment seekers generally tend to have more severe and disabling symptoms and a lower sense of being able to manage their symptoms (low self-efficacy) than general population samples of individuals with fibromyalgia who are not seeking treatment (Box 1) [2]. In an interesting comparative study, the number of lifetime psychiatric diagnoses was significantly higher among fibromyalgia patients compared with

Box 1 Characteristics of Fibromyalgia Treatment Seekers (Based on Kersh [2])

- High pain severity
- Anxiety
- Depression
- High daily stress
- Low level of self-efficacy

(a)

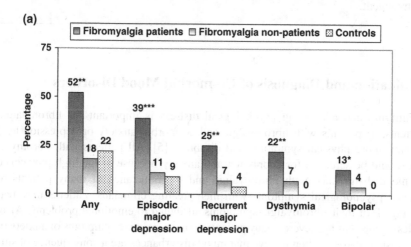

(b)

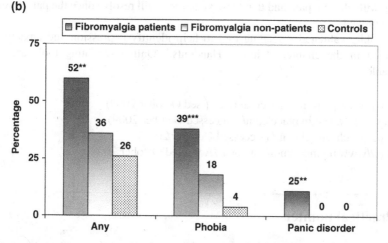

Fig. 2 Psychiatric co-morbidity in fibromyalgia treatment seekers (based on Aaron [3]). (**a**) Mood disorders, (**b**) anxiety disorders. Differences in prevalence between groups were significant: *$P = 0.05$, **$P \leq 0.01$, ***$P \leq 0.001$

fibromyalgia non-patients or controls ($P = 0.002$), although there was no difference between fibromyalgia non-patients and controls (Fig. 2) [3]. Furthermore, patients with personality disorders are more likely to report persistent muscular pain and fibromyalgia and utilize healthcare services, also resulting in overrepresentation of psychiatric disorders among fibromyalgia patient samples [4].

Practical pointer

Mood disorders occur more often in treatment-seeking patients with fibromyalgia, but not in individuals with fibromyalgia who are not seeking treatment.

Evaluation and Diagnosis of Co-morbid Mood Disorders

Identifying and addressing psychological distress is important for fibromyalgia patients, as patients with fibromyalgia and co-morbid anxiety or depression tend to have more physical symptoms and disability [5]. All patients with fibromyalgia should be screened for depression and anxiety because of the high prevalence of mood disturbance with fibromyalgia and the reluctance of many patients to discuss psychological symptoms with their treating clinicians. Patients may fear having all of their fibromyalgia symptoms attributed to emotional problems. Also, unless symptoms are severe, many patients do not recognize symptoms of anxiety or depression. Patients often believe that mood disturbances are a consequence of suffering with chronic pain and that these symptoms will resolve once the pain severity has improved.

Reliable, validated screening tool to help identify depression and anxiety are provided in the chapter "Clinical Handouts." Online screening tools are also available:

- http://www.phqscreeners.com/ (Accessed October 2009)
- http://www.healthyplace.com/ (Accessed October 2009)
- http://psychcentral.com/ (Accessed October 2009)
- http://www.mymoodmonitor.com/ (Accessed October 2009)

Practical pointer

Patients with fibromyalgia should be screened for depression and anxiety.

Self-Efficacy and Locus of Control

Self-efficacy describes a person's beliefs about achieving desired goals. Indeed, self-efficacy has been shown to predict a greater likelihood of engaging in healthy lifestyle practices in patients with fibromyalgia [6]. Furthermore, self-efficacy is linked to reduced pain and disability after fibromyalgia treatment [7].

Locus of control describes beliefs about what causes good or bad things to happen to someone. A belief that one's actions impact his or her own outcome (an internal locus of control) is generally associated with better pain outcome than when individuals believe success is outside of their own control (having an external locus of control) (Table 1).

> **Practical pointer**
>
> An internal locus of control describes a patient's belief that he or she can directly influence his or her own improvement.

Table 1 Locus of control

Locus of control	Beliefs	Example of thoughts
Internal	An internal locus of control results in a healthy view that people can substantially influence their own outcome. People with a strong internal locus of control believe they can control health symptoms through their own behavior and actions. Patients with a strong internal locus of control readily engage in healthy lifestyle behaviors and are compliant with treatment suggestions, understanding their implementation will influence treatment outcome.	When my pain flares, I can use relaxation techniques and exercises to decrease severity. My pain often flares because I skipped exercising or overdid activities. It is important that I keep myself healthy as this will help my fibromyalgia symptoms.
External Powerful others Fate	An external locus of control suggests that an individual can do little to impact his or her own problems, with outcome controlled by powerful others (authority figures, doctors, etc.) or fate. Patients with a strong external locus of control are generally not interested in nor compliant with self-management strategies. They often feel hopeless and helpless and expect improvement will only occur through direct actions by a treating healthcare provider or by chance alone.	There is nothing I can do to keep my pain from getting worse. Nothing that I do helps my fibromyalgia. I just have to wait it out when my pain flares. As soon as my fibromyalgia flares, I have to see the doctor.

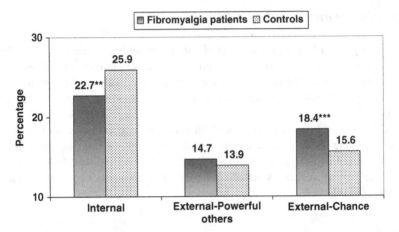

Fig. 3 Locus of control in women with fibromyalgia vs. controls (based on Shuster [8]). Differences in locus of control scores between groups were significant: **$P \le 0.01$, ***$P \le 0.001$

In general, women with fibromyalgia have a higher external locus of control compared with controls (Fig. 3), with an external locus of control significantly correlated with higher ratings of anxiety and depressed mood [8]. In this study, those with fibromyalgia had a significantly lower average score for the more healthy internal locus of control, with a significantly higher score for a chance or fate locus of control. Patients with an external locus of control focused on fate tend to feel helpless and hopeless, believing their outcome is outside of their control and the influence of their healthcare team. In a recent study, individuals with an external locus of control that focused on fate had the greatest likelihood of treatment failure [9]. Once locus of control has been shifted to an internal sense of control, patients are more empowered to participate in and comply with treatment recommendations, as they have a stronger belief that their efforts will directly influence their outcome [10]. Consequently, it is important to understand patients' beliefs about who or what influences their outcomes and help facilitate development of a stronger internal locus of control in those who believe they rely on others or luck to get better.

Practical pointer

Fibromyalgia patients often have an external locus of control, shifting the responsibility for their improvement away from their own actions and onto chance or the actions of others, like their healthcare providers.

A questionnaire for measuring internal and external loci of control is provided in the chapter "Clinical Handouts."

Treatment

When psychological symptoms are mild-moderate in severity, they may be addressed during the course of fibromyalgia treatment. Patients with more severe symptoms will likely need to have psychological symptoms initially addressed in order to subsequently comply with and benefit from other fibromyalgia treatment. Targets for treatment should include improving mood disturbance symptoms and shifting patients to an internal locus of control. While moderately severe symptoms may be managed by general healthcare providers, more severe symptoms may require the expertise of psychologists or psychiatrists. Psychological or psychiatric treatment should occur in concert with rather than in lieu of general fibromyalgia therapy.

Practical pointer

Fibromyalgia patients with considerable psychological distress will need to have treatments directly targeting these symptoms in addition to more general fibromyalgia therapy.

Generally, as patients become engaged in general fibromyalgia treatment, improvements occur in pain, psychological distress, and self-efficacy. This shift in self-efficacy may promote improved treatment compliance, with subsequent enhancement of general treatment efficacy. For this reason, direct treatment of psychological factors should be offered in addition to symptom-relieving therapies to maximize good treatment outcome.

Antidepressants have been consistently shown in clinical trials to improve symptoms of anxiety, depression, and fibromyalgia [11]. Beneficial effects of antidepressants on fibromyalgia are independent of their mood-enhancing properties [11]. Furthermore, in a comparison of treatment outcome with milnacipran between fibromyalgia patients with and without co-morbid depression, greater pain improvement occurred in non-depressed patients, although this was explained by a higher placebo-response rate in the depressed group as opposed to a better analgesic effect in the non-depressed group [11].

Fibromyalgia treatments that focus on self-management techniques also generally result in improved pain, psychological distress, and self-efficacy [12, 13]. Multidisciplinary fibromyalgia treatment that includes educational and/or psychological treatment has been shown to improve pain, mood disturbance, and self-efficacy [14]. Self-efficacy is also improved through Internet-based self-management education [15].

Summary

- Mood disorders affect about two in every three fibromyalgia patients.
- Nearly half of fibromyalgia patients can be diagnosed with a personality disorder.
- Fibromyalgia patients tend to have an external locus of control, believing that improvement depends on luck or the actions of others. Shifting to a stronger internal locus of control is an important treatment target.
- Patients with disabling psychological distress will need treatment directly targeting these symptoms.

References

1. Rose S, Cottencin O, Chouraki V, et al. Study on personality and psychiatric disorder in fibromyalgia. Presse Med. 2009;38:695–700.
2. Kersh BC, Bradley LA, Alarcón GS, et al. Psychosocial and health status variables independently predict health care seeking in fibromyalgia. Arthritis and Rheum. 2001;45:362–71.
3. Aaron LA, Bradley LA, Alarcon GS, et al. Psychiatric diagnoses in patients with fibromyalgia are related to health care-seeking behavior rather than to illness. Arthritis Rheum. 1996;39:436–45
4. Olssøn I, Dahl AA. Personality problems are considerably associated with somatic morbidity and health care utilization. Eur Psychiatry. 2009;24:442–9.
5. White KP, Nielson WR, Harth M, Ostbye T, Speechley M: Chronic widespread musculoskeletal pain with or without fibromyalgia: psychological distress in a representative community adult sample. J Rheumatol. 2002;29:588–94.
6. Beal CC, Stuifbergen AK, Brown A. Predictors of a health promoting lifestyle in women with fibromyalgia syndrome. Psychol Health Med. 2009;14:343–53.
7. Dobkin PL, Liu A, Abrahamowicz M, et al. Predictors of disability and pain six months after the end of treatment for fibromyalgia. Clin J Pain. 2010;26:23–9.
8. Shuster J, McCormack J, Riddell R, Toplak ME. Understanding the psychological profile of women with fibromyalgia syndrome. Pain Res Manag. 2009;14:239–45.
9. Torres X, Collado A, Arias A, et al. Pain locus of control predicts return to work among Spanish fibromyalgia patients after completion of a multidisciplinary pain program. Gen Hosp Psychiatry. 2009;31:137–45.
10. Culos-Reed SN, Brawley LR. Fibromyalgia, physical activity, and daily functioning: the importance of efficacy and health-related quality of life. Arthritis Care Res. 2000;13:343–51.
11. Pae CU, Marks DM, Shah M, et al. Milnacipran: beyond a role of antidepressant. Clin Neuropharmacol. 2009;32:355–63.
12. Menzies V, Taylor AG, Bourguignon C. Effects of guided imagery on outcomes of pain, functional status, and self-efficacy in persons diagnosed with fibromyalgia. J Altern Complement Med. 2006;12:23–30.
13. Rooks DS, Gautam S, Romeling M, et al. Group exercise, education, and combination self-management in women with fibromyalgia: a randomized trial. Arch Intern Med. 2007;167:2192–200.
14. Häuser W, Bernardy K, Arnold B, Offenbächer M, Schiltenwolf M. Efficacy of multicomponent treatment in fibromyalgia syndrome: a meta-analysis of randomized controlled clinical trials. Arthritis Rheum. 2009;61:216–24.
15. Lorig KR, Ritter PL, Laurent DD, Plant K. The internet-based arthritis self-management program: a one-year randomized trial for patients with arthritis or fibromyalgia. Arthritis Rheum. 2008;59:1009–17.

Obesity and Metabolic Syndrome

Key Chapter Points

- About 30% of the general adult population and up to 50% of fibromyalgia patients are obese.
- Obesity in fibromyalgia has been linked to more severe symptom severity.
- Successful weight loss through surgical or non-surgical interventions significantly improves fibromyalgia symptoms.
- Risk for metabolic syndrome is over five times greater in women with fibromyalgia.

Keywords Body mass index · Dyslipidemia · Hyperglycemia

Obesity

According to World Health Organization (WHO) statistics, about 1.6 billion adults were overweight globally in 2005 and at least 400 million were obese [1]. Obesity is a global epidemic, affecting about one in every three to four adults in the United States and Europe (Fig. 1) [2–7]. Obesity also affects Asia, with about one in every four or five adults overweight or obese in China [8].

> **Practical pointer**
>
> One in every three to four adults in the United States and Europe is obese.

Obesity projections are staggering. The WHO projects that 2.3 billion adults will be overweight and over 700 million obese by 2015 [1]. Projections for the United States are shown in Fig. 2 [3]. If these projections prove to be accurate, it is estimated that in the year 2030 in the United States one in every six dollars spent on healthcare will be for health problems attributable to obesity and overweight [3].

D.A. Marcus, A. Deodhar, *Fibromyalgia*, DOI 10.1007/978-1-4419-1609-9_10,
© Springer Science+Business Media, LLC 2011

Case: "Since my diagnosis of fibromyalgia, weight gain has been an added burden. In addition to fibro and the fatigue that goes with it, I also have Hashimoto's thyroiditis and asthma. This makes sticking to an exercise routine difficult at best – either I hurt, I'm already exhausted before I start, I get breathless quickly, or, even with every good effort, the scale budges little at best. There was a time in my life before fibro when a few months of good eating and moderate exercise were all that was needed to keep me in shape. Now, I can eat the same way as before, adopt the same healthy habits, and not see much of a change in weight. It's an uphill struggle."

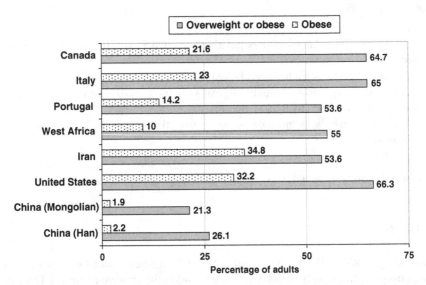

Fig. 1 Worldwide estimates of overweight and obesity (based on Hopman [2], Wang [3], Haijan-Tilaki [4], Abubakari [5], do Carmo [6], Donfrancesco [7], Zhang [8])

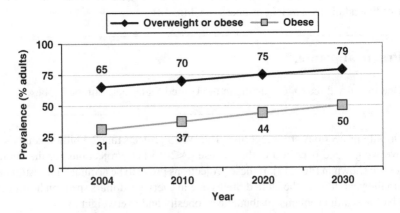

Fig. 2 Obesity projections for the United States (based on Wang [3])

Obesity in Fibromyalgia

Weight status was analyzed in a small sample of 38 fibromyalgia patients (average age 44 years old), using standard body mass index (BMI) weight standards (Table 1) [9]. Average BMI was 30.8 kg/m², with half of the patients obese (Fig. 3). Obesity affected only 30% of a comparable general population sample. Likewise, data from a survey of the fibromyalgia patients through the National Fibromyalgia Association Web site ($N = 1,735$ women, average age $= 47$ years old) reported an average BMI of 30.2 kg/m², with a BMI >25 in 70% and >30 in 43% [10].

> **Practical pointer**
>
> Up to half of fibromyalgia patients are obese.

Table 1 Body mass index

Weight category	BMI (kg/m²)
Normal	<25
Overweight	25–29.9
Obese	≥30

Fig. 3 Weight categories in patients with fibromyalgia (based on Okifuji [9])

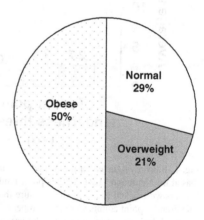

Consequences of Obesity

Obesity has been linked to increased risk for a variety of health conditions, including cardiovascular disease, Type II diabetes, respiratory dysfunction and sleep apnea, osteoarthritis, fatty liver, gallbladder disease, reproductive problems, skin conditions, and cancer and cancer deaths [11]. Obesity also negatively affects fibromyalgia. An evaluation of 100 randomly selected fibromyalgia patients linked BMI to a lower fibromyalgia tender point pain threshold ($P = 0.02$), higher tender point count ($P = 0.01$), physical deconditioning ($P = 0.047$), and poorer quality of life ($P = 0.04$) [12]. Median tender point threshold and tender point counts by weight category are shown in Fig. 4.

Practical pointer

Obese fibromyalgia patients are more sensitive to pain, more likely to be deconditioned, and experience a poorer quality of life.

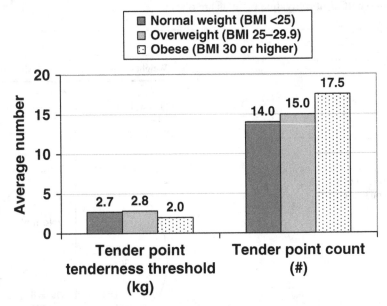

Fig. 4 Fibromyalgia tender points and weight category, based on body mass index (BMI) in kg/m^2 (based on Neumann [12]). Tender point tenderness threshold was assessed using a dolorimeter. Patients were asked to report the pressure that resulted in a change in sensation from pressure to pain. Tender point counts were the number of tender points at which the patients experienced pain when a dolorimeter was applied at 4 kg pressure, with a maximum possible number of 18

Treatment of Obesity

A variety of behaviors have been linked to improved weight loss success (Box 1) [13]. Regularly performing 30 min of exercise results in similar weight loss being achieved when exercise is completed in one long session, two 15-min sessions daily, or three 10-min sessions daily [14]. Furthermore, similar 1-year weight loss occurs with low or moderate caloric restriction diets, suggesting patients should be encouraged to use more easy-to-maintain diets that place fewer restrictions on caloric intake and focus on portion control compared with highly restrictive diets. The most frequently performed surgical options for morbid obesity are laparoscopic Roux-en-Y bypass and laparoscopic gastric banding. A recent literature review concluded that gastric banding was associated with an unacceptably high complication rate, with gastric bypass preferred as the surgical treatment of choice [15].

Box 1 Strategies for Successful Weight Loss (Based on Kruger [13])

- Exercising ≥30 min daily
- Adding physical activity to daily life
- Avoiding over-the-counter diet remedies
- Planning meals
- Counting calories and fat content of foods
- Measuring portion sizes
- Weighing self daily

In an interesting study, the effects of weight reduction on fibromyalgia were evaluated. Overweight and obese fibromyalgia patients enrolled in a 20-week behavioral weight loss course, focusing on dietary management and increased physical activity, including 30 min of daily aerobic exercise [16]. Average weight loss was 9.2 pounds, with a 2-in. reduction in waist circumference (Fig. 5). Pain, disability, and psychological distress were also significantly reduced. Mean depression and anxiety dropped into non-distressed ranges. Although weight was not correlated with symptom severity at baseline, weight loss significantly predicted improvements in fibromyalgia symptoms ($P < 0.05$).

Similarly, a small study in which 10 obese fibromyalgia patients were treated Roux-en-Y gastric bypass showed an average decrease in BMI from 49.4 to 29.7 kg/m^2 ($P = 0.001$) [17]. In conjunction with weight, average pain score (from 1 to 10) decreased from 9.0 to 3.0 ($P = 0.001$) and tender point count decreased from 18.0 to 3.5 ($P = 0.001$). Medication use also decreased in eight patients, with no medication changes in the other two patients.

Practical pointer

Weight loss significantly reduces fibromyalgia symptoms.

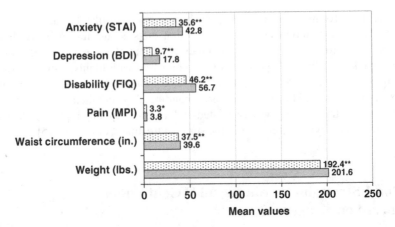

Fig. 5 Effects of weight loss treatment on fibromyalgia (based on Shapiro [16]). All changes from baseline represented significant improvements: *$P < 0.05$, **$P < 0.01$. Weight was measured in pounds and waist circumference in inches. Pain was measured using the Multidimensional Pain Inventory (MPI), which rates pain from 0 to 6 with higher scores representing more severe pain. Disability was rated using the Fibromyalgia Impact Questionnaire (FIQ), which rates fibromyalgia impact from 0 to 100, with higher numbers representing greater negative impact. Depression was measured using the Beck Depression Inventory II (BDI); scores <10 represent no depression and scores of 16–24 represent moderate depression. Anxiety was measured using the State-Trait Anxiety Inventory State Score (STAI); scores >40 signify anxiety

Metabolic Syndrome

Metabolic syndrome includes a constellation of factors linked to increased risk for diabetes and heart disease, including obesity, hypertension, hyperglycemia, and dyslipidemia. The most commonly utilized diagnostic criteria are those provided by the American Heart Association and National Heart, Lung, and Blood Institute [based on the Adult Treatment Panel III (ATP III)] and the International Diabetes Federation, which are nearly identical (Table 2) [18]. The current American Heart Association and National Heart, Lung, and Blood Institute criteria differ from the original ATP III definition, which used a cutoff for hyperglycemia of ≥110 mg/dL. Elevated C-reactive protein levels are a strong predictor of the development of metabolic syndrome, although not part of the diagnostic criteria [19].

A recent meta-analysis of studies using the Adult Treatment Panel III criteria linked the diagnosis of metabolic syndrome to increased risk for cardiovascular disease (relative risk [RR] 1.65, 95% CI 1.38–1.99) and diabetes (RR 2.99, 95% CI 1.96–4.57) [20]. Studies using diagnostic criteria from ATP III and the International Diabetes Federation have shown that both predict increased risk for incident diabetes [21], with risk for coronary artery disease better predicted using the ATP

Table 2 Diagnostic criteria for metabolic syndrome (based on Talim [18])

American Heart Association and National Heart, Lung, and Blood Institute	International Diabetes Federation

At least three of the following:
• Obesity
  – Waist circumference ≥ 102 cm (40 in.) men or ≥88 cm (35 in.) women or
• Dyslipidemia – triglycerides
  – Triglycerides ≥150 mg or dL or patient treated with triglyceride-lowering agent
• Dyslipidemia – HDL cholesterol
  – HDL <40 mg/dL in men or <50 mg/dL in women or patient treated with HDL-elevating agent
• Hypertension
  – SBP ≥130 mg Hg or DBP ≥85 mm Hg or patient treated with blood pressure-lowering agent
• Hyperglycemia
  – Fasting glucose ≥100 mg/dL or treated with glucose-lowering agent
	Obesity, as evidence by increased waist circumference
	PLUS at least two of the following:
	• Dyslipidemia – triglycerides
	  – Triglycerides ≥150 mg or dL or patient treated with triglyceride-lowering agent
	• Dyslipidemia – HDL cholesterol
	  – HDL <40 mg/dL in men or <50 mg/dL in women or patient treated with HDL-elevating agent
	• Hypertension
	  – SBP ≥130 mg Hg or DBP ≥85 mm Hg or patient treated with blood pressure-lowering agent
	• Hyperglycemia
	  – Fasting glucose ≥100 mg/dL (includes diabetes)

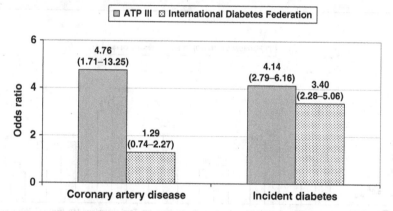

Fig. 6 Prediction coronary artery disease and diabetes by diagnosis of metabolic syndrome, based on Adult Treatment Panel III (ATP III) and International Diabetes Federation criteria (based on Timóteo [22] and Hanley [21]). Odds ratios are shown, with 95% confidence intervals given in parentheses

III criteria, presumably because waist circumference is a less strong predictor than other features (Fig. 6) [22]. Interestingly, while lowering the fasting glucose cutoff requirements from 110 to 100 mg/dL changed the number of people diagnosed with metabolic syndrome, this change did not affect the predictive ability of these criteria for incident diabetes [21].

Metabolic Syndrome in Fibromyalgia

The prevalence of metabolic syndrome was compared in 109 women with fibromyalgia (21–49 years old) and 46 healthy women (21–45 years old) [23]. Over one in every five women with fibromyalgia was diagnosed with metabolic syndrome. Women with fibromyalgia were over 5.5 times more likely to have metabolic syndrome compared with controls. Average scores for metabolic syndrome parameters were all significantly worse in women with fibromyalgia, with the exception of HDL cholesterol which was similar for both groups (Fig. 7). Total and LDL cholesterol were significantly higher among women with fibromyalgia. Due to the high prevalence of metabolic syndrome and elevated cholesterol, triglyceride, glucose, and blood pressure readings in fibromyalgia patients as a group, screening for both metabolic syndrome and the individual features of metabolic syndrome should be part of the routine medical assessment for fibromyalgia patients.

> **Practical pointer**
>
> Metabolic syndrome is over five times more common in women with fibromyalgia.

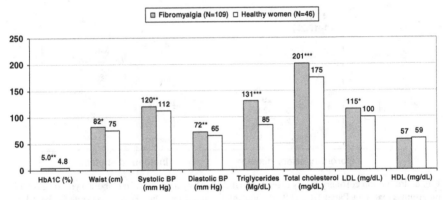

Fig. 7 Metabolic syndrome and cholesterol measurements in women with fibromyalgia and healthy women (based on Loevinger [23]). Age-adjusted significant differences *$P <$ 0.05, ***$P \leq 0.01$, ***$P \leq 0.001$

Treatment of Metabolic Syndrome

Metabolic syndrome is treated with lifestyle modification (including exercise, dietary modifications, and weight reduction) and medication treatment of individual condition components, such as hypertension, diabetes, and dyslipidemia. Specific effects of metabolic syndrome treatment on fibromyalgia symptoms have not been evaluated.

Summary

- Obesity is a global epidemic, affecting one in every three to four adults in Europe and the United States and one in every four to five adults in China.
- Nearly half of fibromyalgia patients are obese.
- Obesity in fibromyalgia patients is linked to a higher tender point count and deconditioning, with lower pain threshold and quality of life.
- Over one in every five women with fibromyalgia has co-morbid metabolic syndrome.
- Monitoring weight and routine screens for blood pressure, hyperglycemia, and dyslipidemia should be part of the general medical assessment for all fibromyalgia patients.

References

1. World Health Organization media centre fact sheets http://www.who.int/mediacentre/factsheets/fs311/en/index.html (Accessed June 2009).
2. Hopman WM, Berger C, Joseph, L, et al. The association between body mass index and health-related quality of life: data from CaMos, a stratified population study. Qual Life Res. 2007;16:1595–1603.
3. Wang Y, Beydoun MA, Liang L, Caballero B, Kumanyika SK. Will all Americans become overweight or obese? estimating the progression and cost of the US obesity epidemic. Obesity. 2008;16:2323–30.
4. Haijan-Tilaki KO, Heidari B. Prevalence of obesity, central obesity and the associated factors in urban population aged 20–70 years, in the north of Iran: a population-based study and regression approach. Obes Rev. 2007;8:3–10.
5. Abubakari AR, Lauder W, Agyemang C, et al. Prevalence and time trends in obesity among adult West African populations: a meta-analysis. Obes Rev. 2008;9:297–311.
6. Do Carmo I, dos Santos O, Camolas J, et al. Overweight and obesity in Portugal: national prevalence in 2003–2005. Obes Rev. 2008;9:11–9.
7. Donfrancesco C, LoNoce C, Brignoli O, et al. Italian network of obesity and cardiovascular disease surveillance: a pilot project. BMC Fam Pract. 2008;9:53.
8. Zhang X, Sun Z, Zheng L, et al. Ethnic differences in overweight and obesity between Han and Mongolian rural Chinese. Acta Cardiol. 2009;64:239–45.
9. Okifuji A, Bradshaw DH, Olson C. Evaluating obesity in fibromyalgia: neuroendocrine biomarkers, symptoms, and functions. Clin Rheumatol. 2009;28:475–8.
10. Jones J, Rutledge DN, Jones KD, Matallana L, Rooks DS. Self-assessed physical function levels of women with fibromyalgia: a national survey. Women's Health Issues. 2008;18:406–12.
11. Brown WV, Fujikoa K, Wilson PW, Woodworth KA. Obesity: why be concerned? Am J Med. 2009;122:S4–11.
12. Neumann L, Lerner E, Glazer Y, Bolotin A, Shefer A, Buskila D. A cross-sectional study of the relationship between body mass index and clinical characteristics, tenderness measures, quality of life, and physical functioning in fibromyalgia patients. Clin Rheumatol. 2008;27:1543–7.

13. Kruger J, Blanck HM, Gillespie C. Dietary and physical activity behaviors among adults successful at weight loss maintenance. Int J Behav Nutr Phys Act. 2006;3:17.
14. Schmidt WD, Biwer CJ, Kalscheuer LK. Effects of long versus short bout exercise on fitness and weight loss in overweight females. J Am Coll Nutr. 2001;20:494–501.
15. Guller U, Klein LV, Hagen JA. Safety and effectiveness of bariatric surgery: Roux-en-Y gastric bypass is superior to gastric banding in the management of morbidly obese patients. Patient Saf Surg. 2009;3:10.
16. Shapiro JR, Andersen DA, Danoff-Burg S. A pilot study of the effects of behavioral weight loss treatment on fibromyalgia symptoms. J Psychosom Res. 2005;59:275–82.
17. Saber AA, Boros MJ, Manci T, et al. The effect of laparoscopic Roux-en-Y gastric bypass on fibromyalgia. Obes Surg. 2008;18:652–5.
18. Talim S, Tai ES. The relevance of the metabolic syndrome. Ann Acad Med Singapore. 2009;38:29–33.
19. Bo S, Rosato R, Cinccone G, et al. What predicts the occurrence of the metabolic syndrome in a population-based cohort of adult healthy subjects? Diabetes Metab Res Rev. 2009;25: 76–82.
20. Ford ES. Risks for all-cause mortality, cardiovascular disease, and diabetes associated with the metabolic syndrome: a summary of the evidence. Diabetes Care. 2005;28:1769–78.
21. Hanley AG, Karter AJ, Williams K, et al. Prediction of type 2 diabetes mellitus with alternative definitions of the metabolic syndrome. The Insulin Resistance Atherosclerosis Study. Circulation. 2005;112:3713–21.
22. Timóteo A, Santos R, Lima S, et al. Será que a definição de síndroma metabólica pela *International Diabetes Federation* melhora a capacidade preditora para doença coronéria e do espessamento da íntima-média carotídea? Rev Port Cardiol. 2009;28:173–81.
23. Loevinger BL, Muller D, Alonso C, Coe CL. Metabolic syndrome in women with chronic pain. Metabolism. 2007;56:87–93.

Part III
Treatment

Published Recommendations

Key Chapter Points

- Evidence-based recommendations for the treatment of fibromyalgia are available.
- Published guidelines cover both medication and non-medication treatments.
- Evidence-based recommendations provide guidelines to help direct treatment selection for individual patients.

Keywords Exercise · Evidence-based · Guidelines · Medication · Non-medication

Case presentation

Dr. M. recently completed his family practice residency before joining a large clinical practice. "Sometimes I think the senior partners send all of their difficult pain patients to us junior staff. This week, I saw three women with fibromyalgia and I don't know what to do for them. I know there are a number of treatments for fibromyalgia, but what I've tried just doesn't seem to make a big impact. Before I get to an effective treatment, my patients get so frustrated that I think they begin to wonder if I really know what I'm doing! I wish there was someone to tell me what really worked and where I should start with treatment."

A wide range of medication and non-medication treatments have been tested in patients with fibromyalgia. No individual or combination of therapies has provided definitive symptomatic resolution, with benefits often modest and inconsistent among studies. Consequently, several evidence-based guidelines have been published to help provide guidance for treatment selection. A recent review compared fibromyalgia guidelines published from 2005 to 2008 [1]. Differences in how data were collected and evaluated and the composition of the panels analyzing available data likely led to some of these differences among recommendations. In general, however, guidelines supported treating patients with both medication and

D.A. Marcus, A. Deodhar, *Fibromyalgia*, DOI 10.1007/978-1-4419-1609-9_11,
© Springer Science+Business Media, LLC 2011

non-medication therapies, including tricyclic antidepressants, aerobic exercise, and cognitive-behavioral therapy. Three of the most recent evidence-based guidelines in the English literature, each published in 2008, are reviewed below.

Ottawa Panel Evidence-Based Exercise Guidelines

A Canadian panel of experts, including medical personnel and epidemiologists with extensive experience in developing evidence-based guidelines, evaluated data from comparative controlled trials assessing the role of exercise in the treatment of fibromyalgia [2, 3]. Effective exercise included fitness exercise and strength training. Benefits from strengthening occurred in both middle-aged and elderly patients. Fitness exercises result in improvements in pain, quality of life, and endurance/function in fibromyalgia patients. Strengthening exercises improved pain, quality of life, muscle strength, and mood. A broad range of improvement with exercise was demonstrated in a small study in which 34 women with fibromyalgia were randomized to treatment with aerobic, proprioceptive, and strengthening exercises or a no-exercise control group for 12 weeks [4]. Exercise was performed three times weekly. There was no change in pain or quality of life in the control group. In contrast, women assigned to exercise experienced a 29% reduction in pain ($P = 0.01$) and a 93% improvement in quality of life ($P = 0.007$). Benefits were lost during a subsequent de-training period, highlighting the benefits of active exercise. This study demonstrated several important features of exercise in fibromyalgia:

- Pain reduction with exercise, though significant, is modest.
- Quality of life benefits exceed pain reduction, highlighting the importance of assessing additional measures besides simply pain levels when determining efficacy.
- Exercise needs to continue long term, as benefits will likely be lost if exercise is discontinued.

Practical pointer

Aerobic exercise is expected to modestly decrease pain, with greater improvements in quality of life.

Based on the studies included in the Ottawa Panel review, the following specific exercise recommendations can be given to patients:

- Fitness exercise
  - Effective fitness exercise includes pool or land-based aerobic exercise.
  - Fitness exercises should be performed three times weekly, 60 min per session.

- Strength training

  - A strengthening program is more beneficial for fibromyalgia patients than flexibility training.
  - Strengthening should be performed twice weekly for 60 min per session.

Practical pointer

Fibromyalgia treatment should include 60 min of daily exercise, alternating aerobics and strength training.

European League Against Rheumatism (EULAR)

The European League Against Rheumatism (EULAR) task force, comprised of a multidisciplinary team of 19 individuals from 11 European countries, developed evidence-based fibromyalgia treatment guidelines [5]. Their recommendations were formed after reviewing clinical trials specifically evaluating treatments in patients with fibromyalgia diagnosed using the American College of Rheumatology 1990 criteria [6]. Recommendations were generated for both medication and non-medication therapy. Recommendations were based on assessing improvements in pain (based on visual analogue pain severity scores) and function (based on the Fibromyalgia Impact Questionnaire). Additional outcome measures that might have been used by studies were not considered.

Practical pointer

Fibromyalgia treatment should include a combination of medication and non-medication therapies.

EULAR endorsed multidisciplinary treatment, combining medication and non-medication treatments (Box 1). Medication recommendations included the use of tramadol, antidepressants, pregabalin, dopamine agonist pramipexole [7], and intravenous serotonin antagonist tropisetron. Data supporting the use of these and other medications for the treatment of fibromyalgia are detailed in the chapter "Medication Treatments". EULAR supported the exercise recommendations endorsed by the Ottawa Panel (above) and further supported inclusion of warm water therapy, based on consistently beneficial data shown in numerous studies. Soothing heated water therapy temporarily reduces pain symptoms and may facilitate exercise therapy. Controlled studies evaluating the benefits of exercise treatment

> ## Box 1 European League Against Rheumatism (EULAR) Recommendations for Fibromyalgia Treatment (Based on Carville 2008 [5])
>
> - Treatment should include both medication and non-pharmacological therapies
> - Effective medications
>
>   - Tramadol
>   - Antidepressants
>   - Pregabalin
>   - Tropisetron
>   - Pramipexole
>   - Possibly simple analgesics (paracetamol/acetaminophen or weak opioids)
>   - Strong opioids and corticosteroids are not recommended
>
> - Effective non-pharmacological treatments
>
>   - Heated pool treatment with or without exercise
>   - Aerobic exercise
>   - Strength training
>   - Cognitive-behavioral therapy
>   - Possibly relaxation, rehabilitation, physical therapy, and psychological support

in waist-high warm water (33°C) or a control showed that water-based exercise conducted for 1 h, three times weekly resulted in a 29% reduction in pain, as well as improved muscle strength and quality of life short term.[55] Warm water exercise has also been shown to improve cognitive function in addition to reducing pain symptoms in fibromyalgia patients [8]. Long-term studies show that warm water exercise for 8 months is cost-effective, with improvements noted in treated patients compared with controls of 8% for pain and 20% for physical function [9, 10]. Additional support was provided for utilization of psychological pain management techniques, especially cognitive-behavioral therapy.

EULAR intends to update their recommendations every 5 years, which will provide up-to-date guidelines, based on the most currently available clinical trials.

> ## Practical pointer
>
> Medications with good evidence for efficacy in fibromyalgia include tramadol, antidepressants, pregabalin, pramipexole, and tropisetron.

German Interdisciplinary Association of Pain Therapy

Because of a stronger focus on medication compared with non-medication thera-pies of previously published guidelines, such as those developed by EULAR [5], the German Interdisciplinary Association of Pain Therapy sought to develop more com-prehensive recommendations that would include a more interdisciplinary focus [11]. Their evidence-based recommendations were developed through literature review and consensus from a panel of 15 medical experts and 2 patients representing large fibromyalgia self-help groups. This panel developed recommendations for both medication and non-drug therapies (Table 1). These recommendations provided a detailed analysis of a wide range of non-drug treatments and a strong recommen-dation for patient education and interdisciplinary or multidisciplinary treatment. Multidisciplinary treatment was recommended to include at least one psycholog-ical intervention and one exercise component. Their recipe for optimal first-line treatment of disabling fibromyalgia included the combination of:

- Patient education
- Cognitive-behavioral therapy
- Aerobic exercise
- Amitriptyline
- Treatment of co-morbid conditions

Table 1 German Interdisciplinary Association of Pain Therapy recommendations for fibromyalgia treatment (Based on Häuser 2008 [11])

Treatment category	Strongly recommended	Moderately recommended	Not recommended
Non-drug	Patient education Aerobic exercise Cognitive-behavioral therapy with relaxation	Massage	Acupuncture Dietary manipulation
Medication	Antidepressants (tricyclic amitriptyline; SNRI duloxetine; SSRI fluoxetine and paroxetine)	Tramadol alone or in combination with acetaminophen	SSRI citalopram Anesthetic injections or blocks

SNRI=serotonin norepinephrine reuptake inhibitor; SSRI=selective serotonin reuptake inhibitor

Limitations of Current Guidelines

While published recommendations provide excellent road maps for treatments to consider in fibromyalgia patients, it is important to recognize that additional treat-ments that may be beneficial may not have been reviewed because of a lack of appropriately designed studies. Furthermore, many of the studies utilized for determining these evidence-based recommendations included only short-term outcome measures. While short-term efficacy is important, long-term data are needed to help identify: (1) which treatments provide long-term efficacy and (2) how long treatments need to be utilized once patients have achieved symptomatic reduction. These guidelines also fail to highlight the need to individualize treatment regimens for each patient, based on patient symptom complexes, co-morbidities, and treatment tolerability. Clinicians must recognize that these recommendations are general guidelines rather than treatment mandates for the individual patient.

Summary

- Up-to-date guidelines for treating fibromyalgia were published in 2008 by the Canadian and European expert panels.
- Evidence-based guidelines recommend utilization of both medication and non-medication therapies.
- Recommendations for medications include tramadol, antidepressants, pregabalin, pramipexole, and tropisetron.
- Recommendations for non-medication treatments include patient education, cognitive-behavioral therapy, and fitness and strengthening exercises.

References

1. Häuser W, Thiene K, Turk DC. Guidelines on the management of fibromyalgia syndrome – a systematic review. Eur J Pain. 2010;14:5–10.
2. Brosseau L, Wells GA, Tugwell P, et al. Ottawa panel evidence-based clinical practice guidelines for aerobic fitness exercises in the management of fibromyalgia: part 1. Phys Ther. 2008;88:857–71.
3. Brosseau L, Wells GA, Tugwell P, et al. Ottawa panel evidence-based clinical practice guidelines for strengthening exercises in the management of fibromyalgia: part 2. Phys Ther. 2008;88:873–86
4. Gusi N, Tomas-Carus P, Häkkinen A, Häkkinen K, Ortega-Alonso A. Exercise in waist-high warm water decreases pain and improves health-related quality of life and strength in the lower extremities in women with fibromyalgia. Arthritis Rheum. 2006;55:66–73.
5. Carville SF, Arendt-Nielsen S, Bliddal H, et al. EULAR evidence-based recommendations for the management of fibromyalgia syndrome. Ann Rheum Dis. 2008;67:536–41.
6. Wolfe F, Smythe HA, Yunus MB, et al. The American College of Rheumatology 1990 criteria for the classification of fibromyalgia. Arthritis Rheum. 1990;33:160–72.
7. Holman AJ, Myers RR. A randomized, double-blind, placebo-controlled trial of pramipexole, a dopamine agonist, in patients with fibromyalgia receiving concomitant medications. Arthritis Rheum. 2005;52:2495–505.
8. Munguía-Izquierdo D, Legaz-Arrese A. Exercise in warm water decreases pain and improves cognitive function in middle-aged women with fibromyalgia. Clin Exp Rheumatol. 2007;25:823–30.
9. Gusi N, Tomas-Carus P. Cost-utility of an 8-month aquatic training for women with fibromyalgia: a randomized controlled trial. Arthritis Res Ther. 2008;10:R24.

10. Tomas-Carus P, Gusi N, Häkkinen A, et al. Eight months of physical training in warm water improves physical and mental health in women with fibromyalgia: a randomized controlled trial. J Rehabil Med. 2008;40:248–52.
11. Häuser W, Arnold B, Eich W, et al. Management of fibromyalgia syndrome – an interdisciplinary evidence-based guideline. Ger Med Soc. 2008;6:doc 14.

Medication Treatments

Key Chapter Points

- Effective medications should be expected to reduce fibromyalgia pain and other symptoms by about 30%.
- Because symptomatic reduction is modest to moderate, medications should generally be used as part of a more comprehensive pain management program rather than as monotherapy.
- Both SNRI antidepressants and neuromodulating antiepileptics have analgesic properties and produce clinically meaningful fibromyalgia improvement.
- Both antidepressants and antiepileptics significantly improve pain, sleep, and quality of life, while antidepressants additionally reduce fatigue and depressed mood.
- A wide range of drugs are currently being studied as potential new treatments for fibromyalgia.

Keywords Antidepressant · Antiepileptic · Emerging therapies · Meaningful improvement · Tramadol

Case

*I've been treating patients in a primary care practice for the last eight years. I've tried several antidepressants and pregabalin for my fibromyalgia patients – and nothing really seems to work. Their pain may decrease by a third or half, but they still have a lot of pain and other symptoms – even when I'm using the doses that have been shown to be effective in the clinical trials. How come these treatments never really seem to help **my** patients?*

Medication treatments for fibromyalgia ideally reduce pain by 30–50%, although this level of improvement is not achieved by most patients.

D.A. Marcus, A. Deodhar, *Fibromyalgia*, DOI 10.1007/978-1-4419-1609-9_12,
© Springer Science+Business Media, LLC 2011

Consequently, medications are best used in conjunction with effective non-drug treatments rather than as monotherapy to maximize symptomatic reduction in fibromyalgia patients. Both healthcare providers and patients need to have realistic expectations for the amount of relief they might anticipate from their fibromyalgia medications. Effective drug treatments can be expected to result in modest symptomatic reduction; marked resolution of pain and other symptoms is not a realistic goal for most fibromyalgia medications.

Data from a survey of almost 2,600 people with fibromyalgia showed that, while medication use is high, the benefit achieved from medications is generally only moderate at best (Fig. 1) [1]. As will be seen throughout this chapter, studies evaluating medications for fibromyalgia consistently support only modest symptomatic relief even for the most effective medications. Understanding the limitations from medication therapy can help healthcare providers develop realistic treatment goals when treating with fibromyalgia medications. In general, fibromyalgia treatments can be divided into those with high, moderate, and minimal efficacy, with most patients ideally being treated with those medications with higher anticipated efficacy. Although considered to be first-line medication treatments for fibromyalgia, effective treatments are not expected to result in complete resolution of all fibromyalgia symptoms. This chapter will review data from drugs approved for fibromyalgia treatment, drugs not specifically approved for fibromyalgia but commonly used in clinical practice, and emerging therapies to help facilitate determining reasonable treatment strategies and expectations for benefit.

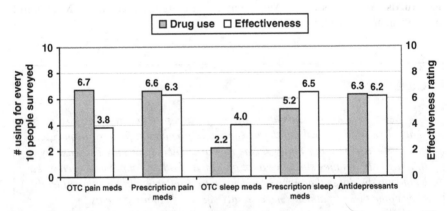

Fig. 1 Use and perceived effectiveness of medications for fibromyalgia (based on Bennett [1]). Drug use is shown as the number of people using each drug category for every 10 people surveyed. Effectiveness was rated on a scale from 0 = no help to 10 = helpful

Effective Medications

Both antidepressants and neuromodulating antiepileptics have demonstrated significant efficacy for reducing symptoms in fibromyalgia patients. Drugs that have been approved by the Food and Drug Administration (FDA) for the specific treatment of fibromyalgia include the antidepressants duloxetine [Cymbalta] and milnacipran [Savella] and the antiepileptic pregabalin [Lyrica]. Other antidepressants and antiepileptics may also produce good symptomatic relief. Although effective drugs have been proven to significantly reduce fibromyalgia symptoms, it is important to understand that anticipated symptomatic reduction is generally modest to moderate. Consequently, these therapies are best used in conjunction with effective non-drug treatments (such as aerobic exercise and psychological pain management techniques) rather than as monotherapy to maximize patient improvement.

Practical pointer

Drugs that are the most effective for treating fibromyalgia are antidepressants and neuromodulating antiepileptics.

Antidepressants

Similar to using antidepressants for treating other chronic pain conditions, antidepressants are likewise effective in patients with fibromyalgia whether or not they have co-morbid depression [2]. Recent functional MRI data support a more comprehensive analgesic effect from antidepressants in fibromyalgia patients, rather than simply benefit from mood improvement [3]. Furthermore, a recent study showed that treatment with milnacipran produced both reduced pain sensitivity and a parallel activation of brain descending inhibitory pathways in fibromyalgia patients, additionally supporting direct analgesic benefit from antidepressants [3]. A recent meta-analysis of antidepressant therapy for fibromyalgia identified significant improvements in pain, fatigue, sleep disturbance, mood, and health-related quality of life with antidepressants [4]. There were differences among different classes of antidepressants, with a broader range of symptoms addressed by the tricyclic antidepressant amitriptyline and SNRIs (Table 1). While monoamine oxidase inhibitors (MAOIs) have shown benefit for pain reduction in fibromyalgia, they are generally not recommended as fibromyalgia treatment because MAOIs have not effectively treated other fibromyalgia symptoms and they are difficult to manage outside of specialty practices.

Practical pointer

Antiepileptics improve a more narrow range of fibromyalgia symptoms than antidepressants. Symptoms that improve significantly with neuromodulating antiepileptics include pain, sleep, and quality of life.

Table 1 Strong evidence supporting antidepressants for improving fibromyalgia symptoms (based on Häuser [4])

| Symptom | Antidepressant category | | | |
	Tricylic (amitriptyline)	SNRIs (duloxetine and milnacipran)	SSRIs (fluoxetine and paroxetine)	MAOIs (moclobemide and pirindole)
Pain	Effective ($P < 0.001$)	Effective ($P < 0.001$)	Effective ($P = 0.04$)	Effective ($P = 0.03$)
Fatigue	Effective ($P = 0.003$)	Not effective	Not effective	Not effective
Sleep	Effective ($P < 0.001$)	Effective ($P < 0.001$)	Not effective	Not effective
Depressed mood	Not effective	Effective ($P = 0.001$)	Effective ($P = 0.02$)	Not effective
Quality of life	Effective ($P = 0.04$)	Effective ($P < 0.001$)	Effective ($P = 0.03$)	Data not available

MAOI = monoamine oxidase inhibitor; SNRI = serotonin norepinephrine reuptake inhibitor; SSRI = selective serotonin reuptake inhibitor

Serotonin and Norepinephrine Reuptake Inhibitors (SNRIs)

Among antidepressants, serotonin and norepinephrine reuptake inhibitors (SNRIs) offer the best efficacy and tolerability for fibromyalgia (Table 2) [5, 6]. Both duloxetine and milnacipran have proven efficacy in randomized, blinded, controlled studies. Interestingly, duloxetine is more effective in female fibromyalgia patients,

Table 2 Comparison of antidepressant effectiveness for fibromyalgia (based on Littlejohn [5])

Effectiveness	Medication
Good	Duloxetine [Cymbalta] Milnacipran [Savella]
Moderate	Amitriptyline [Elavil]
Inconsistent	Venlafaxine [Effexor] Fluoxetine [Prozac]
Ineffective	Citalopram [Celexa]

with minimal benefit in males [7]. Tolerability is superior with SNRIs compared with tricyclic antidepressants, with nausea the most common side effect with SNRIs. Long-term safety and efficacy with duloxetine has been demonstrated in clinical trials monitoring patients for 12 months of treatment [8, 9].

Pooled data from four randomized, controlled clinical trials testing duloxetine for fibromyalgia were used to determine which specific symptoms needed to get better for patients to experience clinically meaningful improvement [10]. Pain and symptoms that interfered with the ability to work were highly correlated with patient global improvement, while function, depression, anxiety, and fatigue were moderately correlated with global improvement. Independent predictors of patient impression of global improvement included measures of pain, function, and anxiety. These data support the need to target improvements in function, fatigue, and mood, in addition to pain, to achieve the most meaningful patient improvement.

> ### Practical pointer
>
> Global improvement is independently predicted by reductions in pain, functional disability, and anxiety, making these each important treatment targets.

Clinically meaningful improvement with duloxetine was also evaluated using data pooled from randomized clinical trials treating either fibromyalgia or neuropathic pain [11]. An average change in pain of 34% resulted in a corresponding rating of "much better" or "very much better" on the Patient Global Impression of Improvement Scale. Pain reduction of >50% was consistently linked to a global improvement rating of "very much better." Reduction in Pain Scores [using a 0 (no pain) to 10 (excruciating pain) rating scale] of three points was linked to a global impression of "much" or "very much better" and a reduction of four points was linked to "very much better" (Table 3).

Treatment efficacy can be evaluated by considering those important targets to achieve the clinically meaningful improvement described above. Pooled data from two clinical trials treating women with fibromyalgia with 60 mg duloxetine twice daily showed improvements across a broad range of symptoms, although substantial pain reduction occurred in only about one in three women (Table 4) [12]. Pooled data from five clinical trials revealed that the most common AEs with duloxetine

Table 3 Pain reduction targets to achieve clinically meaningful relief (based on Farrar [11])

Change in 0–10 Pain Severity Rating Scale	Global impression of at least "much better"	Global impression of "very much better"
Change in score	−3	−4
Percent change	−34	−51

Table 4 Changes in efficacy measures with duloxetine (based on Arnold [12])

Efficacy measure change vs. pre-treatment	Duloxetine 60 mg twice daily		Between-treatment P-value
	Duloxetine (N = 326)	Placebo (N = 212)	
Pain severity [0–10 severity scale]			
Raw score	−2.07	−0.94	<0.001
≥30% pain reduction	39%	19%	<0.001
≥50% pain reduction	30%	13%	<0.001
Fibromyalgia impact questionnaire			
Total score	−14.29	−7.01	<0.001
Interference with work	−2.02	−0.92	<0.001
Tiredness	−1.57	−0.92	<0.01
Tender point threshold	0.30	0.01	<0.001

were nausea, headache, dry mouth, insomnia, fatigue, constipation, diarrhea, and dizziness [13]. Discontinuations due to AEs occurred for 20% with duloxetine and 12% with placebo.

Likewise, a randomized clinical trial evaluating milnacipran for fibromyalgia reported ≥30% pain improvement plus a global impression of "much better" or "very much better" in 27% of patients treated with milnacipran 200 mg daily, 26% with milnacipran 100 mg daily, and 19% with placebo [14]. Improvements in individual symptoms are shown in Table 5. The most commonly reported AEs were constipation, hyperhidrosis, hot flush, vomiting, heart rate increased, dry mouth, palpitations, and hypertension. Discontinuations due to AEs occurred for 27% with milnacipran 200 mg, 20% with milnacipran 100 mg, and 10% with placebo.

Table 5 Changes in efficacy measures with milnacipran (based on Mease [14])

Efficacy measure	Milnacipran 200 mg daily (N = 441)	Milnacipran 100 mg daily (N = 224)	Placebo (N = 223)
Pain severity			
≥30% pain reduction	52.8%***	56.2%*	40.2%
≥50% pain reduction	37.0%*	34.7%	26.2%
Fibromyalgia Impact Questionnaire			
Total score	−16.7	−17.7	−15.0
Multidimensional Fatigue Inventory	−5.8*	−5.0	−3.4

Between-treatment differences were significant: $^*P < 0.05$, $^{***}P = 0.001$

Tricyclics

Amitriptyline is the tricyclic that has been most extensively evaluated for fibromyalgia. In five randomized, clinical trials, low-dose amitriptyline (25 mg at bedtime) resulted in significant improvements in a variety of fibromyalgia symptoms, including pain, sleep disturbance, and fatigue after 6–8 weeks of treatment [15]. Reductions in average pain score (on an 11-point severity scale) in the two 8-week studies reporting pain score change were −2.1 and −3.5 points. A single 12-week study with 25 mg amitriptyline included in this review failed to show benefit. Four studies evaluating 50 mg amitriptyline dosing showed no benefit over placebo, except for significantly better sleep in one of the two studies that measured sleep disturbance as an outcome measure.

Selective Serotonin Reuptake Inhibitors (SSRIs)

Selective serotonin reuptake inhibitors (SSRIs) are generally less effective for reducing fibromyalgia symptoms than SNRIs or tricyclics. For example, a randomized, controlled 12-week trial with paroxetine ($N = 116$) showed no difference between paroxetine and placebo for pain relief, with an average decrease in pain of 1.2 points on an 11-point pain severity scale [16]. Improvements in Fibromyalgia Impact Questionnaire (FIQ) total scores of at least 25 and 50%, respectively, were achieved by 57 and 26% with paroxetine vs. 33 and 14% with placebo. Similarly, a smaller, 12-week, randomized, controlled study ($N = 60$) showed ≥25% improvement in FIQ pain and total scores, respectively, in 56 and 32% with fluoxetine vs. 15% with placebo for both scores [17]. Concerns have been raised about increased suicide risk with SSRIs, especially in younger patients with major depression.

Antiepileptics

Pregabalin [Lyrica] was approved by the FDA for the treatment of fibromyalgia in 2007. Gabapentin [Neurontin] has also demonstrated efficacy in decreasing pain, disability, and sleep disturbance in fibromyalgia patients in a randomized, double-blind, placebo-controlled clinical trial [18]. Dizziness and somnolence are common side effects with both pregabalin and gabapentin, affecting about one in three treated patients. In addition, the FDA recently announced a warning about increased risk of suicide among patients using some antiepileptic drugs, including pregabalin and gabapentin [19].

A recent meta-analysis of randomized, controlled clinical trials evaluating pregabalin or gabapentin for fibromyalgia treatment showed that treating with these neuromodulating antiepileptics resulted in significant improvement for a range of symptoms ($P<0.001$ for each symptom) [20]:

- Pain
- Sleep
- Quality of life

There was no significant benefit for fatigue, anxiety, or depressed mood. This meta-analysis showed a mean reduction in pain (on an 11-point pain severity scale) of 0.95–2.06 with pregabalin and 0.72–1.40 with placebo.

Practical pointer

Antidepressants result in significant improvement in a broad range of fibromyalgia symptoms, including pain, fatigue, sleep, mood, and quality of life.

Using an area-under-the-curve analysis, the average responses among fibromyalgia patients treated with pregabalin or placebo in a recent, 14-week, randomized clinical trial were 34% for pregabalin 600 mg/day, 31% for pregabalin 450 mg/day, 29% for pregabalin 300 mg/day, and 21% for placebo [21]. All doses of pregabalin resulted in significantly more pain reduction than with placebo ($P < 0.05$).

Sleep Therapy

Endogenous neurochemical gamma-hydroxybutyric acid or GHB is involved in sleep regulation. GHB gained notoriety in the 1990s when it was used as a nutritional supplement, sleep aid, and club drug associated with date rape. In 2002, a medical compound based on GHB called sodium oxybate [Xyrem] was approved for the treatment of narcolepsy with cataplexy. Phase II trials in fibromyalgia began in 2005.

Sodium oxybate is administered by providing half of the nightly dose at bedtime, with the second half administered 2.5–4 h later. An 8-week, randomized, double-blind, placebo-controlled trial ($N = 188$) with sodium oxybate 4.5 g or 6 g/day or placebo resulted in a $\geq 30\%$ and 50% reduction in pain, respectively, for 39–41% and 28–29% with sodium oxybate vs. 20 and 14% with placebo ($P = 0.02$ for both doses for 30%, $P = 0.05$ for 6 g, and 0.08 for 4.5 g for 50%) [22]. Improvement in FIQ was twice as good with sodium oxybate as placebo ($P \leq 0.02$). Data from a subsequent, 14-week controlled trial similarly treating fibromyalgia patients with a total nighttime dose of 4.5 or 6 g sodium oxybate or placebo showed significant improvements in pain, fatigue, and sleep disturbance (Fig. 2) [23]. The most commonly reported side effects with sodium oxybate are headache, nausea, dizziness, and somnolence. Patients with severe sleep apnea, severe hypertension, and congestive heart failure should avoid using sodium oxybate.

Tight regulations for prescribing sodium oxybate have been used to minimize possible diversion and unwanted abuse with sodium oxybate for recreational purposes. Sodium oxybate prescribers need to be certified and all prescriptions are

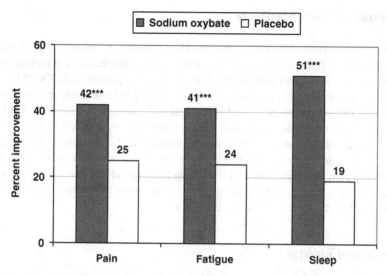

Fig. 2 Efficacy of sodium oxybate for fibromyalgia symptoms (based on Mease [14]). Pain and fatigue were both measured using Visual Analogue Scales. Sleep was measured using the Jenkins Sleep Scale. Improvements were similar for both doses of sodium oxybate, so results have been averaged here. Significant improvements were seen in each symptom vs baseline: ***$P < 0.001$

distributed through a central pharmacy to minimize diversion. Implementation of these regulations has resulted in relatively few cases of drug misuse or abuse [24].

Moderate Efficacy Medications

The combination analgesic tramadol 37.5 mg and acetaminophen 325 mg has been shown to significantly improve pain, function, and quality of life in patients with fibromyalgia [25, 26]. In a double-blind, randomized, placebo-controlled study ($N = 313$), average pain severity decreased by 26% in fibromyalgia patients taking tramadol plus acetaminophen (average dose 4.0 ± 1.8 pills daily) for 3 months vs. a decrease of 10% with placebo ($P < 0.001$) [25]. The number of tender points at baseline was 16 ± 2 in both treatment groups, decreasing to 13 ± 5 tender points with tramadol plus acetaminophen and 14 ± 4 tender points with placebo ($P = 0.04$). Fibromyalgia Impact Score decreased by 19% with tramadol and placebo vs. 9% with placebo ($P = 0.008$).

A recently published animal study showed that combining treatment with the antidepressant milnacipran and the analgesic tramadol was more significantly effective in reducing mechanical hyperalgesia in an animal model of fibromyalgia produced by acidic saline injections into gastrocnemius muscles than treatment with either therapy alone [27]. This potentiation of anti-hyperalgesic effect from combination therapy supports the clinical practice of using individual medications as part of a more comprehensive treatment program rather than as monotherapy [28].

Minimal Efficacy Medications

Analgesics have limited benefit for fibromyalgia patients. A review of four placebo-controlled trials testing nonsteroidal anti-inflammatory medications in patients with fibromyalgia failed to find superiority of analgesics over placebo [29]. Opioids offer limited value for fibromyalgia pain. The United States FDA recently recommended decreasing the maximum permitted individual acetaminophen dose from 1,000 to 650 mg and the total daily allowed acetaminophen dose from 4,000 to 3,250 mg to reduce unintentional acetaminophen-related toxicity, including potential liver damage [30]. Because acetaminophen is included in a wide range of over-the-counter and prescription analgesic products, including both opioid and non-opioid preparations, total daily dose used by patients can become quite high when all sources of acetaminophen are included in this calculation.

Practical pointer

Analgesics are generally ineffective for reducing fibromyalgia pain.

Despite the lack of efficacy of analgesics for treating fibromyalgia, a recent survey of 434 women with fibromyalgia revealed that nonsteroidal anti-inflammatory drugs were the second most common category of drugs used after antidepressants, which were used by half of the participants. Analgesics, however, were used by a surprising number of patients:

- Nonsteroidal anti-inflammatory drugs – 30%
- Opioid analgesics – 21%
- Other analgesics (e.g., aspirin and acetaminophen) – 18%

Healthcare providers need to educate their patients about the generally poor response expected from analgesics for fibromyalgia patients, to minimize excessive use of these medications. Analgesics are best reserved for the treatment of severe, intermittent flares rather than as routine fibromyalgia therapy.

General Fibromyalgia Medication Recommendations

General medication recommendations treating fibromyalgia are provided in Table 6. Guidelines for treatment include the following:

- Fibromyalgia treatment will require comprehensive treatment approaches that will include non-medication and, in many cases, additional medication therapy. Medication monotherapy is generally not effective for disabling fibromyalgia.
- Medication treatment should be initiated with first-line therapy, unless otherwise contraindicated.

Table 6 Medication recommendations for fibromyalgia

First-line drugs	Second-line drugs	Third-line drugs
• SNRIs: duloxetine [Cymbalta] 60 mg once or twice a day and milnacipran [Savella] 50–100 mg twice a day • Pregabalin [Lyrica] 450 mg daily	• Sodium oxybate (Xyrem 4.5–6 g nightly)[a] • Tricyclic antidepressants: amitriptyline [Elavil] 25 mg at bedtime • Gabapentin [Neurontin] 400–800 mg three times daily • Tramadol 37.5 mg plus acetaminophen 325 mg [Ultracet] every 6 h, as needed	• SSRIs: fluoxetine [Prozac] 10–60 mg/day and paroxetine [Paxil] 20–40 mg/day

SNRI = serotonin norepinephrine reuptake inhibitor; SSRI = selective serotonin reuptake inhibitor.

[a]Despite good efficacy, sodium oxybate is considered to be second tier treatment due to stricter regulations with prescribing and monitoring patients

- Symptomatic improvement from medications is often modest at best. Effective medications should be expected to reduce symptoms by about 30%.
- A pain reduction of about 30% or a decrease in pain score of 3 on an 11-point Pain Severity Scale (0 = no pain; 10 = excruciating pain) is considered to be clinically meaningful.

It is important to recognize that many patients will not experience significant benefit from drugs with proven efficacy, even with those drugs that have been rigorously tested and approved for the treatment of fibromyalgia by regulatory agencies. This point was highlighted in the previously mentioned meta-analysis of randomized studies testing pregabalin and gabapentin for fibromyalgia [20]. A total of 8.5 patients needed to be treated for one patient to achieve at least a 30% decrease in pain severity (number-needed-to-treat [NNT] analysis). Likewise, NNT to achieve the more stringent criteria of ≥50% reduction in pain for duloxetine in one clinical trial was seven patients [31]. A similar analysis of data from three duloxetine trials, including the one described above [27] calculated a NNT for ≥50% reduction in pain with duloxetine of 6.4 patients [32]. These data highlight that, even when using treatments with proven efficacy, not all patients will benefit. Clinically meaningful symptomatic improvement will be maximized by using these treatments within a comprehensive treatment program.

Emerging Therapies

Medications tested as possible treatment for fibromyalgia with results available in the literature include the noradrenergic antidepressant reboxetine [33], narcolepsy

Table 7 Emerging therapies for fibromyalgia

Reference	Medication	Study design	Outcome
Krell (2005)	Reboxetine 8 mg/day	Case report $N = 3$	Improvements in pain, functioning, mood, and fatigue
Schwartz (2007)	Modafinil average dose 162 mg/day	Retrospective chart review $N = 98$	28% reduction in fatigue ($P < 0.001$)
Toda (2008)	Neurotropin 4 tablets per day (dose not specified)	Case report $N = 1$	Subjective pain decreased by half
Hidalgo (2007)	Quetiapine 25–100 mg/day	Open-label, 12-week trial $N = 30$	No effect on pain FIQ decreased 16% ($P < 0.001$)
Cuarecasas (2007)	Growth hormone 0.0125 mg/kg/day subcutaneously	Randomized, open-label 1-year treatment of usual care with or without growth hormone $N = 24$	Number of tender points decreased by 63% with growth hormone vs. 6% with usual care ($P = 0.0001$). FIQ improved by 46% with growth hormone vs. 9% with usual care ($P < 0.05$)
Schafranski 2009	Five sequential intravenous 2% lidocaine infusions with rising dosages (2–5 mg/kg)	Open-label, 1-month trial $N = 23$	Significant improvements after 5 and 30 days, respectively, in pain [16% ($P = 0.01$) and 12% ($P = 0.05$)] and FIQ (13% at both time points [$P \leq 0.04$]). Two patients (9%) experienced a 50% reduction in pain after the fifth infusion

FIQ = Fibromyalgia Impact Questionnaire

treatment modafinil [Provigil] [34], antipsychotic quetiapine [Seroquel] [35], nerve growth modulator neurotropin [NT in Japan] [36], growth hormone [37], and intravenous lidocaine [38] (Table 7). Sodium oxybate and neurotropin have also demonstrated at least anecdotal efficacy for treating chronic fatigue syndrome [39, 40].

Phase II clinical trials have also been completed with the antiepileptic lacosamide [Vimpat] and transdermal dopamine agonist rotigotine [Neupro], although data are not yet available in the literature. Additional drugs currently involved in clinical trials for the treatment of fibromyalgia include

- Hypnotic eszopiclone [Lunesta] – Phase IV
- Narcolepsy treatment armodafinil [Nuvigil] – Phase IV
- Calcitonin – Phase IV
- Atypical antipsychotic quetiapine [Seroquel] – Phase IV
- Nerve growth modulator neurotropin [NT in Japan] – Phase II

Summary

- Effective fibromyalgia medications should be expected to reduce pain by about one-third.
- Clinically meaningful pain reduction is generally achieved when pain decreases by at least three points on an 11-point pain scale (0 = no pain, 10 = excruciating pain) or pain decreases by about 30%.
- Effective medications for reducing fibromyalgia symptoms include SNRI antidepressants duloxetine and milnacipran, neuromodulating antiepileptic pregabalin, and narcolepsy therapy sodium oxybate.
- The range of fibromyalgia symptoms improved by antidepressants is more comprehensive than symptoms improved with antiepileptics.
- A wide range of medications are currently being investigated for efficacy against fibromyalgia symptoms.

References

1. Bennett RM, Jones J, Turk DC, Russell IJ, Matallana L. An internet survey of 2,596 people with fibromyalgia. BMC Musculoskeletal Disorders. 2007;8:27.
2. Arnold LM, Hudson JI, Wang F, et al. Comparisons of the efficacy and safety of duloxetine for the treatment of fibromyalgia in patients with versus without major depressive disorder. Clin J Pain. 2009;25:461–8.
3. Mainguy Y. Functional magnetic resonance imagery (fMRI) in fibromyalgia and the response to milnacipran. Hum Psychopharmacol. 2009;24:S19–23.
4. Häuser W, Bernardy K, üçeyler N, Sommer C. Treatment of fibromyalgia syndrome with antidepressants: a meta-analysis. JAMA. 2009a;301:198–209.
5. Littlejohn GO, Guymer EK. Fibromyalgia syndrome: which antidepressant drug should we choose. Curr Pharm Des. 2006;12:3–9.
6. Arnold LM. Duloxetine and other antidepressants in the treatment of patients with fibromyalgia. Pain Med. 2007;8:S63–74.
7. Arnold LM, Lu Y, Crofford LJ, et al. A double-blind, multicenter trial comparing duloxetine with placebo in the treatment of fibromyalgia patients with or without major depressive disorder. Arthritis Rheum. 2004;50:2974–84.
8. Mease PJ, Russell J, Kajdasz DK, et al. Long-term safety, tolerability, and efficacy of duloxetine in the treatment of fibromyalgia. Semin Arthritis Rheum. 2010;39:454–64.
9. Chappell AS, Littlejohn G, Kajdasz DK, et al. A 1-year safety and efficacy study of duloxetine in patients with fibromyalgia. Clin J Pain. 2009;25:365–75.

10. Hudson JI, Arnold LM, Bradley LA, et al. What makes patients with fibromyalgia feel better? Correlations between Patient Global Impression of Improvement and changes in clinical symptoms and function: a pooled analysis of 4 randomized placebo-controlled trials of duloxetine. J Rheumatol. 2009;36:2517–22.

11. Farrar JT, Pritchett YL, Robinson M, Praakash A, Chappell A. The clinical importance of changes in the 0 to 10 numeric rating scale for worst, least, and average pain intensity: analyses of data from clinical trials of duloxetine in pain disorders. J Pain. 2010;11:109–18.

12. Arnold LM, Pritchett YL, D-Souza DN, et al. Duloxetine for the treatment of fibromyalgia in women: pooled results from two randomized, placebo-controlled clinical trials. J Womens Health. 2007;16:1145–56.

13. Choy EH, Mease PJ, Kajdasz DK, et al. Safety and tolerability of duloxetine in the treatment of patients with fibromyalgia: pooled analysis of data from five clinical trials. Clin Rheumatol. 2009;28:1035–44.

14. Mease PJ, Clauw DJ, Gendreau RM, et al. The efficacy and safety of milnacipran for treatment of fibromyalgia. a randomized, double-blind, placebo-controlled trial. J Rheumatol. 2009;36:398–409.

15. Nishishinya B, Urrútia G, Walitt B, et al. Amitriptyline in the treatment of fibromyalgia: a systematic review of its efficacy. Rheumatology. 2008;47:1741–6.

16. Patkar AA, Masand PS, Krulewicz S, et al. A randomized, controlled, trial of controlled release paroxetine in fibromyalgia. Am J Med. 2007;120:448–54.

17. Arnold LM, Hess EV, Hudson JI, et al. A randomized, placebo-controlled, double-blind, flexible-dose study of fluoxetine in the treatment of women with fibromyalgia. Am J Med. 2002;112:191–7.

18. Arnold LM, Goldenberg DL, Stanford SB, et al. Gabapentin in the treatment of fibromyalgia: a randomized, double-blind, placebo-controlled, multicenter trial. Arthritis Rheum. 2007;56:1336–44.

19. http://www.fda.gov/cder/drug/InfoSheets/HCP/antiepilepticsHCP.htm (Accessed February. 2008).

20. Häuser W, Bernardy K, üçeyler N, Sommer C. Treatment of fibromyalgia syndrome with gabapentin and pregabalin – a meta-analysis of randomized controlled trials. Pain. 2009b;145:69–81.

21. Cappelleri JC, Bushmakin AG, Zlateva G, Sadosky A. Pain responder analysis: use of area under the curve to enhance interpretation of clinical trial results. Pain Pract. 2009;9:348–53.

22. RussellIJ, Perkins AT, Michalek JE. Sodium oxybate relieves pain and improves function in fibromyalgia syndrome: a randomized, double-blind, placebo-controlled, multicenter clinical trial. Arthritis Rheum. 2009;60:299–309.

23. Mease PJ, Swick TJ, Alvarez-Horine S, et al. Sodium oxybate improves fatigue, sleep disturbance, and PGIC in fibromyalgia: results from a phase III, 14-week controlled trial. Presented at the 2009 ACR/ARHP Annual Scientific Meeting, October 16–21, 2009, Philadelphia, PA.

24. Wang YG, Swick TJ, Carter LP, Thorpy MJ, Benowitz NL. Safety overview of poatmarketing and clinical experience of sodium oxybate (Xyrem): abuse, misuse, dependence, and diversion. J Clin Sleep Med. 2009;5:365–71.

25. Bennett RM, Kamin M, Karim R, Rosenthal N. Tramadol and acetaminophen combination tablets in the treatment of fibromyalgia pain: a double-blind, randomized, placebo-controlled study. Am J Med. 2003;114:537–45.

26. Bennett RM, Schein J, Kosinski MR, et al. Impact of fibromyalgia pain on health-related quality of life before and after treatment with tramadol/acetaminophen. Arthritis Rheum. 2005;53:519–27.

27. Kim SH, Song J, Mun H, Park KU. Effect of the combined use of tramadol and milnacipran on pain threshold in an animal model of fibromyalgia. Korean J Intern Med. 2009;24:139–42.

28. Häuser W, Arnold B, Eich W, et al. Management of fibromylagia syndrome – an interdisciplinary evidence-based guideline. Ger Med Soc. 2008;6:doc 14.

29. Lautenschläger J. Present state of medication therapy in fibromyalgia syndrome. Scand J Rheumatol. 2000;29:32–6.
30. Krenzelok EP. The FDA acetaminophen advisory committee meeting – what is the future of acetaminophen in the United States? The perspective of a committee member. Clin Toxicol (Phila). 2009;47:784–9.
31. Russell IJ, Mease PJ, Smith TR, et al. Efficacy and safety of duloxetine for treatment of fibromyalgia in patients with or without major depressive disorder: Results from a 6-month, randomized, double-blind, placebo-controlled, fixed-dose trial. Pain. 2008;136:432–44.
32. Sultan A, Gaskell H, Derry S, Moore RA. Duloxetine for painful diabetic neuropathy and fibromyalgia pain: systematic review of randomised trials. BMC Neurology. 2008;8:29.
33. Krell HV, Leuchter AF, Cook IA, Abrams M. Evaluation of reboxetine, a noradrenergic antidepressant, for the treatment of fibromyalgia and chronic low back pain. Psychosomatics. 2005;46:379–84.
34. Schwartz TL, Rayancha S, Rashid A, et al. Modafinil treatment for fatigue associated with fibromyalgia. J Clin Rheumatol. 2007;13:52.
35. Hidalgo J, Rico-Villademoros F, Calandre EP. An open-label study of quetiapine in the treatment of fibromyalgia. Prog Neuropsychopharmacol Biol Psychiatry. 2007;31:71–7.
36. Toda K, Tobimatsu Y. Effiacy of neurotropin in fibromyalgia: a case report. Pain Med. 2008;9:460–3.
37. Cuatrecasas G, Riudavets C, Güell MA, Nadal A. Growth hormone as concomitant treatment in severe fibromyalgia associated with low IGF-1 serum levels. A pilot study. BMC Musculoskelet Disord. 2007;8:119.
38. Schafranski MD, Malucelli T, Machado F, et al. Intravenous lidocaine for fibromyalgia syndrome: an open trial. Clin Rheumatol. 2009;28:853–5.
39. Moldofsky H. The significance of the sleeping-waking brain for the understanding of widespread musculoskeletal pain and fatigue in fibromyalgia syndrome and allied syndromes. Joint Bone Spine. 2008;75:397–402.
40. Toda K, Kimura H. Efficacy of neurotropin in chronic fatigue syndrome: a case report. Efficacy of neurotropin in chronic fatigue syndrome: a case report. Hiroshima J Med Sci. 2006;55:35–7.

Non-medication Treatments

Key Chapter Points

- The most effective non-medication therapies are aerobic and strengthening exercises and cognitive- and operant-behavioral therapies.
- Performing exercises in a pool may facilitate benefits.
- Modest benefits may be achieved with manual therapy, yoga, and relaxation techniques.
- Acupuncture is generally ineffective for fibromyalgia.
- Lifestyle modifications, including smoking cessation, sleep regulation, and weight management, are important for improved general health, with some fibromyalgia-specific symptom benefits also expected.

Keywords Aerobic · Cognitive-behavioral · Hydrotherapy · Operant-behavioral · Sleep · Smoking

Case presentation

"After years of having fibromyalgia, I have learned what works for me and what doesn't. Still, sometimes flares happen and you deal with them as best as you can. Most days, I can push through my flares using a variety of pain management techniques and go to work. Every so often, I see my limit has been reached and accept it for that particular day, remembering tomorrow is always another day with another chance to reevaluate. Working with my doctor, we've been able to figure out which flares will likely be killer flares that won't get better on their own over the course of a day. When this happens, I've learned to take a sick day to focus on my flare techniques and maybe see my therapist for manual therapy. I've found that it's better to take off the occasional day and improve rather than suffering through days of agony."

D.A. Marcus, A. Deodhar, *Fibromyalgia*, DOI 10.1007/978-1-4419-1609-9_13,
© Springer Science+Business Media, LLC 2011

Table 1 Frequency and effectiveness of common non-medication treatments (based on Bennett [1])

Treatment	% Patients utilizing	Effectiveness rating[a]
General treatments		
Rest	86	6.3
Prayer	57	6.0
Walking	64	4.6
Psychological treatments		
Relaxation	47	5.1
Distraction	80	4.7
Cognitive-behavioral therapy	8	4.3
Hypnosis	3	2.5
Physical treatments		
Heat	74	6.3
Massage	43	6.1
Pool therapy	26	6.0
Stretching	62	5.4
Non-aerobic exercise	24	5.1
Chiropracty	30	5.1
Aerobic exercise	32	5.0
Cold	30	4.8
Physical therapy	24	4.7
Acupuncture	15	4.5
Strengthening	18	4.3

[a]Effectiveness rated from 0 = not helpful to 10 = helpful

The frequency with which fibromyalgia patients utilize different non-medication treatments and their reported success is shown in Table 1 [1]. These data clearly show that, while fibromyalgia patients often do utilize non-medication treatments, they do not necessarily select those therapies that have been shown to be most helpful for fibromyalgia symptoms. The most effective therapies for fibromyalgia include aerobic exercise and psychological pain management techniques. These therapies have also been most rigorously tested in well-designed clinical trials. As described below, exercise and strengthening exercises are the most beneficial physical treatments; however, according to the survey, more fibromyalgia patients use less effective heat, stretching, and massage [1]. Likewise, although cognitive-behavioral therapy is one of the most effective psychological techniques, less than 10% of fibromyalgia patients use these techniques [1].

A variety of complementary and alternative therapies have been evaluated, although most randomized trials have fairly low-quality methodology, limiting interpretation [2]. The best evidence for beneficial complementary medicine has been for hydrotherapy, for which significant benefit has been shown in multiple, well-designed clinical trials [2]. In a recent study, 19 fibromyalgia patients were treated with tanning beds three times weekly [3]. For the first 2 weeks of the study, patients were acclimated to the tanning beds, spending time in both the actual ultraviolet tanning bed and the non-ultraviolet control bed. After these 2 weeks, patients were randomized to 6 weeks of treatment with either the ultraviolet or the control bed. There was no significant improvement in pain, fatigue, or disability with either condition and no between-treatment differences.

Physical Treatments

Physical treatments that typically improve most types of chronic pain are often ineffective for patients with fibromyalgia. Consequently, it is important to develop a specific fibromyalgia exercise treatment program rather than utilizing the typical stretching exercises and myofascial techniques that are often beneficial for other common chronic pain conditions.

Exercise

The benefits from exercise for fibromyalgia were recently evaluated in a Cochrane Database review of 34 studies testing 47 exercise interventions [4]. Their review resulted in several general recommendations:

- Aerobic exercise should be performed for a total of at least 20 min daily, 2–3 days per week. Exercise may be divided into two 10-min sessions.
  - Aerobic exercise should be gradually increased to achieve a moderate intensity level.
  - Moderate intensity aerobic exercise improves physical function and well-being, without substantial improvement in pain.
- Strength training should be performed 2–3 days per week, with at least 8–12 repetitions per exercise.

  - Strength training improves pain, mood, and well-being, but not physical function.

Specific expectations of improvement from training are shown in Table 2. Although numerical improvements are superior with strengthening compared with aerobic exercise, it is important to recognize that the quality of data available for assessing aerobic exercise is better than that for strengthening training. Consequently, treatment with both aerobic exercise and strength training is recommended.

Practical pointer

Effective fibromyalgia exercise includes aerobic exercise and strength training.

Table 2 Expected outcome from exercise compared with not exercising (based on Busch [4])

Outcome measure	Aerobic exercise	Strengthening training
Well-being (using 0–100 point scale)	+7 points	+41 points
Pain (using 0–10 point scale)	−1.3 points	−4.9 points
Tender points	Increase tender point threshold by 0.23 kg/cm^2	Two fewer positive tender points

Stretching exercise and myofascial therapy, which are generally very helpful for non-fibromyalgia pain, are typically not effective for fibromyalgia. A recent small study (N=20) randomized fibromyalgia patients to stretching exercises plus kinesio-therapy or myofascial physiotherapy, with training sessions provided twice weekly for 150 min per week for 12 weeks [5]. Patients in both treatment groups experienced increases in flexibility at treatment endpoint that persisted when re-assessed after 3 months. Improvement in fibromyalgia symptoms, however, was modest and temporary. At the end of treatment, tender point count and disability, respectively, decreased by 17% ($P = 0.005$) and 42% ($P = 0.01$) with stretching and 16% (not significant) and 22% ($P=0.04$) with myofascial therapy; however, when assessed 3 months later, benefits were lost.

Practical pointer

Traditional chronic pain physical therapy, focusing on stretching and myofascial treatment, is ineffective for fibromyalgia.

Hydrotherapy

Therapeutic hydrotherapy may include balneotherapy (drinking or bathing in medicinal water), bathing in warm or cold water or mud, and spa therapy (drinking or bathing in thermal or mineral waters). A meta-analysis of 10 randomized trials evaluating hydrotherapy for 446 fibromyalgia patients showed significant reductions in pain ($P < 0.0001$) and quality of life ($P = 0.008$) [6]. Average time of treatment was 240 min. Interpretation of these data, however, is limited due to the relatively small number of patients included in each individual study. The largest study included in this review randomized patients already being treated with medication therapy to either their usual medications ($N = 40$) or medications plus the addition of 12 mud packs and 12 thermal baths administered over 2 weeks ($N = 40$) [7]. There was no significant change in the usual care group, while the addition of 2 weeks of

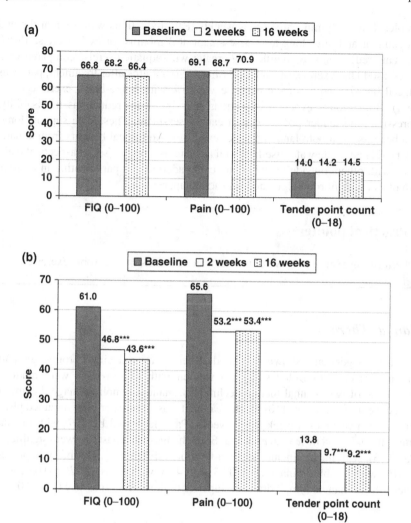

Fig. 1 Effects of hydrotherapy (based on Fioravanti [7]). (**a**) Usual care alone, (**b**) usual care plus hydrotherapy. Pain was measured using a Visual Analogue Scale. Ranges for each measure are shown in *parentheses*. FIQ = Fibromyalgia Impact Questionnaire. Significant changes vs. baseline: ***$P < 0.001$

hydrotherapy to usual care resulted in significant improvements in pain, disability, and tender point count ($P < 0.001$) (Fig. 1). Perhaps most importantly, improvements realized at the conclusion of hydrotherapy were maintained 14 weeks later.

Aquatic therapy provides the benefits of exercise in the soothing and supportive environment of warm pool water. In a recent controlled study, 63 fibromyalgia patients were randomized to 5 weeks of treatment with group aquatic exercise or a home-based land exercise program [8]. In both cases, exercises were to be completed over 60 min, three times weekly. Pain reductions were seen at the end of treatment and after long-term assessment at 3 months for both exercise therapies. Pain reduction was significantly greater with aquatic exercise compared with home-based land exercise at each assessment. Six months after treatment, pain was reduced by 37% with aquatic exercise vs. 16% with home-based exercise ($P = 0.004$). Both groups experienced similar and significant reductions in disability, depression, and tender point count at each assessment. These data support long-term benefits from both land and water exercises. Additional benefits from aquatic may be related to the water itself, as well as benefits from the social aspects of exercising with others outside of the home, camaraderie from participating in a group with others with fibromyalgia, and instructor supervision.

> **Practical pointer**
>
> Performing exercises in water may enhance benefits from aerobic exercise.

Manual Therapy

Massage has generally shown only modest benefit for reducing fibromyalgia pain [9]. In a recent, controlled study, 50 women with fibromyalgia were randomized to one of two manual therapy techniques: manual lymph drainage therapy or connective tissue massage [10]. Each treatment was administered by a trained physiotherapist, five times a week, for 3 weeks. Pain decreased by 79% with manual lymph drainage and 60% with massage. Both changes from baseline were significant ($P < 0.05$), with no significant between-treatment differences. Disability improved by 61% with lymph drainage ($P < 0.05$) and 42% with massage ($P < 0.05$), with benefits from manual lymph drainage superior to those from massage ($P = 0.01$).

Yoga

In a small, open-label study, 33 fibromyalgia patients were treated with weekly yoga for 8 weeks, with each session lasting about 50 min [11]. Pain and disability improved during treatment, with continued benefits 1 month after completing treatment. In this study, pain remained decreased by about 20% and disability by about 30% when patients were re-assessed 4–6 weeks after completing treatment.

Work Simplification and Pacing

Although not specifically tested in clinical trials, an occupational therapy assessment, followed by suggestions for using appropriate ergonomics, work simplification, and pacing techniques can be important steps for minimizing fibromyalgia-related disability. Occupational therapists can address the variety of factors that affect maintaining activity levels and work commitments [12], including specific work duties and the ability to adjust or modify work tasks to reduce pain flares, as well as interfacing with the employer to facilitate necessary modifications to ensure the least impact on both work productivity and symptom severity. In a recent analysis, fibromyalgia patients who chose to self-pace their activities rather than eliminating tasks or requesting help to perform chores or tasks were less disabled than those who avoided physical activities or asked others for assistance [13]. Therefore, patients should be educated about scheduling, pacing, and work simplification to minimize fibromyalgia-related disability.

Acupuncture

The effect of acupuncture on fibromyalgia pain was recently evaluated in a systematic review and meta-analysis of six randomized trials treating 323 subjects [14]. There was no significant improvement in pain severity. Consequently, acupuncture is not routinely recommended for fibromyalgia.

Psychological Treatments

Case presentation

Psychological pain management techniques help patients accept their fibromyalgia symptoms and develop proactive techniques to minimize pain interference, as well as specific skills for reducing pain flares. Patients learning these techniques develop a healthy attitude about their pain symptoms that leads to more positive and effective responses when symptoms increase.

Fibromyalgia patient Sheryl S. eloquently describes the importance of developing effective coping strategies: "The attitude we choose in dealing with fibromyalgia is as important as the treatments we pursue. To live well with fibromyalgia, you need to accept the diagnosis and understand that, while you didn't cause yourself to get fibromyalgia, there are many things you can do to minimize how much it interferes with your life. Whether your doctor says you are doing too much or too little, the implication is that somehow YOU are the cause, when fibromyalgia really isn't your fault. Blaming ourselves doesn't help and is detrimental to progress in treatment. I find it's best to say, 'It is what it is; I didn't cause it, it's not my fault, but how can I improve my life from here?' "

In contrast to traditional psychoanalytic therapy, which aims to determine emotional reasons *why* symptoms occur, effective psychological pain management strategies focus on modifying behaviors and emotions that can occur as a *consequence* of chronic pain. A recent review of psychological treatments for fibromyalgia pain evaluated data from 32 randomized controlled studies [15]. The most robust pain improvement occurred with cognitive-behavioral therapy (CBT) and operant-behavioral therapy (OBT) group treatments, which resulted in a 50% improvement in pain in 42–65% of treated patients. Furthermore, benefits were often maintained for 6–24 months after completing treatment. A cost analysis showed an annual increase in both hospital costs (+$1,906 per patient) and primary care costs (+$442 per patient) after standard medical treatment for fibromyalgia vs. annual decreases in both hospital (–$3,933 per patient) and primary care (–$1,840 per patient) costs with CBT or OBT treatment. Relaxation monotherapy did not show benefit, and hypnotherapy and a writing intervention expressing traumatic experiences resulted in only mild benefits. Psychoanalysis is generally not used as general treatment for fibromyalgia.

Practical pointer

The most effective pain management techniques for fibromyalgia are cognitive-behavioral therapy and operant-behavioral therapy.

Cognitive-Behavioral Therapy and Operant-Behavioral Therapy

CBT focuses on replacing maladaptive thoughts and behaviors with effective coping strategies and adaptive behaviors designed to reduce pain perception and interference, improve functional status, and boost self-efficacy. For example, patients who tend to catastrophize about their pain report greater physical impairment and more disability [13]. With CBT, patients are taught to replace catastrophizing ("This pain will never get better. I'm doomed to spend the day in bed.") with adaptive coping messages ("I need to pace my activities better and add in some extra flare management techniques when my pain increases.")

OBT seeks to identify pain behaviors, such as expressing pain symptoms, grimacing, moaning, and limping, which serve to elicit unwanted positive pain reinforcement from others. For example, when family and friends notice pain behaviors, they may become excessively solicitous, reinforce avoiding activities, increase catastrophic thinking, and encourage treating pain with increased medications or doctor visits. OBT encourages increasing activity, taking medications on a time-contingent basis rather than in response to pain symptoms, and teaching significant others to reinforce positive behaviors.

In a controlled study, 125 fibromyalgia patients were randomized to CBT, OBT, or an attention-placebo control [16]. Each treatment consisted of 15 weekly 2-h sessions conducted in groups of five patients. Patients learning CBT were also trained in relaxation techniques. Although there were no significant differences immediately post-treatment, long-term benefit was significantly better for both CBT and OBT compared with the control for pain, disability, affective distress, and number of physician visits (Fig. 2). The only outcome difference between CBT and OBT was a significantly lower number of physician visits at 12 months for patients treated with OBT ($P = 0.01$). A clinically meaningful benefit was defined as improving by $\geq 50\%$. Clinically meaningful improvement in pain and physical disability, respectively, occurred for 45 and 38% with CBT, 54 and 58% with OBT, and 5 and 8% with placebo [17].

Combining relaxation with CBT has also shown benefit in a small study ($N = 14$) [18]. In this study, patients were treated for 6 weeks, with outcome data obtained 1 month after completing treatment. Significant improvements occurred for pain (45% reduction, $P = 0.03$), disability (35% reduction on the Fibromyalgia Impact Questionnaire, $P < 0.01$), and self-efficacy (29% improvement, $P = 0.02$).

Lifestyle Modifications

Adopting healthy general lifestyle habits, like avoiding nicotine, regulating the sleep cycle, and maintaining a healthy weight, is important for overall well-being and good health. Interestingly, these treatments also offer benefits for fibromyalgia-specific symptoms. Therefore, healthy lifestyle changes should be included in every fibromyalgia treatment plan.

Smoking Cessation

A recent survey reported that one in every four fibromyalgia patients smokes [19]. Consuming nicotine-containing products alters several important neurochemicals that influence pain activity, including endorphins [20], serotonin, norepinephrine, and dopamine [21]. Nicotine, consequently, negatively enhances pain sensitivity. A study of experimental pain showed that chronic nicotine exposure in rodents sensitized nerves and increased the development of painful hypersensitivity after nerve injury [22]. Humans with pain conditions are also negatively impacted by smoking. For example, individuals currently or previously smoking at least 20 cigarettes per day have 50–70% higher risk for experiencing moderate–severe pain and pain affecting more body locations than individuals who never smoked [23].

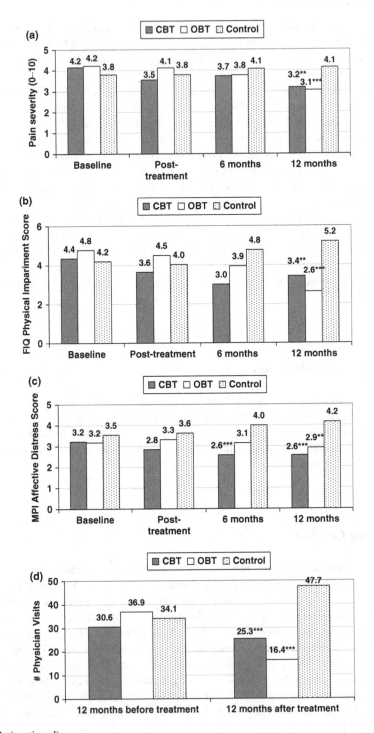

Fig. 2 (continued)

Nicotine also affects medication use and efficacy. Current and former smokers have an increased risk of analgesic use compared with non-smokers [24]. In addition to using more analgesics, smokers reap less pain-relieving benefit from analgesics than non-smokers. Opioid concentration and pain severity were evaluated in 100 healthy adults with non-specific chronic low-back pain [25]. Smokers required higher doses of hydrocodone and reported higher pain scores post-treatment than non-smokers (Fig. 3). Despite greater opioid intake, opioid blood levels (in this case, hydrocodone) were actually lower in smokers compared with non-smokers.

Practical pointer

While nicotine likely did not cause fibromyalgia symptoms, patients should be educated that smoking will likely:

- Increase pain sensitivity
- Increase the need for pain killers
- Reduce the analgesic potency of pain killers

Nicotine has also been linked to increased fibromyalgia symptoms. In an interesting study, 984 consecutive fibromyalgia patients were evaluated, 15% of whom were smokers [26]. Although tender point counts were similar between groups (mean of 16 for each group), Fibromyalgia Impact Questionnaire (FIQ) total score and subscores for physical impairment, work interference, pain, restful sleep, stiffness, anxiety, and depression were all significantly more impaired ($P<0.05$) among patients who used tobacco (Fig. 4). Average, best, and worst pain were similarly significantly more severe among tobacco users ($P<0.05$).

Practical pointer

Nicotine use significantly increases pain and other fibromyalgia-related symptoms.

Fig. 2 (continued) Benefits of psychological pain management treatments for fibromyalgia (based on Thieme [16]). (**a**) Pain severity: at 12 months, pain was significantly better for both CBT (**$P = 0.01$) and OBT (***$P < 0.001$) compared with control, (**b**) physical impairment: at 12 months, impairment was significantly less for both CBT (**$P = 0.004$) and OBT (***$P = 0.001$) compared with control, (**c**) affective distress: at 6 months, distress was significantly less with CBT (***$P < 0.001$): at 12 months, distress was significantly less for both CBT (***$P < 0.001$) and OBT (**$P = 0.004$) compared with control, (**d**) number of physician visits in the 12 months before treatment and 12 months after treatment: at 12 months, distress was significantly less for both CBT and OBT (***$P < 0.001$ for both) compared with control. FIQ = Fibromyalgia Impact Questionnaire; MPI = West Haven-Yale Multidimensional Pain Inventory

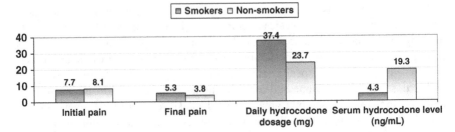

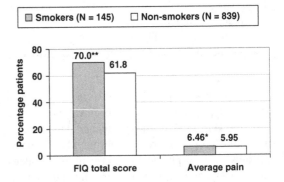

Fig. 3 Relationship between smoking and pain and analgesia (based on Ackerman [25]). Smokers used at least one pack of cigarettes per day. All patients were treated with monotherapy with hydrocodone, with a maximum daily dosage of 40 mg for 4 weeks. Pain is rated on a 0 (no pain) to 10 (excruciating pain) severity scale. Significant between groups differences occurred for final pain, hydrocodone dosage, and hydrocodone levels ($P < 0.05$)

Fig. 4 Comparison of fibromyalgia symptoms in smokers vs. non-smokers (based on Weingarten [26]). Pain was rated on a $0 =$ no pain to $10 =$ severe pain scale. Significant differences between groups: $*P = 0.01$, $**P < 0.001$

Sleep Hygiene

The benefits of behavioral treatment of sleep dysfunction were evaluated in an inter-esting study in which 42 fibromyalgia patients with chronic insomnia complaints were randomly treated with CBT, sleep hygiene, or usual care [27]. Patients treated with either CBT or sleep hygiene received basic education about sleep cycles and sleep needs. Patients assigned to CBT were also instructed to adopt a standard rise time, leave the bed during extended periods when unable to sleep, use the bed only for sleep and sex, and avoid daytime naps. Patients in the sleep hygiene group were instructed to limit caffeine and alcohol consumption, engage in regular moderate exercise, have a light bedtime snack, and keep the bedroom dark, quiet, and cool. Sleep logs revealed a nearly 50% reduction in nighttime wake time with CBT com-pared with a 20% reduction with sleep hygiene and 4% reduction with usual care (Fig. 5). Sleep was considered to be clinically improved for 57% treated with CBT, 17% with sleep hygiene, and none with usual care. Mental health quality of life was significantly improved with both CBT and sleep hygiene compared with usual care ($P = 0.02$), while pain scores were significantly better with sleep hygiene but not CBT ($P = 0.02$). Interestingly, an evaluation of those patients treated with sleep

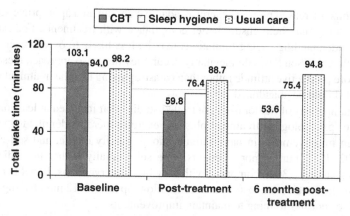

Fig. 5 Change in total time awake at night with CBT and sleep hygiene (based on Edinger [27]). Analysis of covariance showed a significant between-group difference ($P = 0.005$), with a paired comparison showing significantly better reduction in nocturnal wake time with CBT (but not sleep hygiene) compared with usual care

hygiene who experienced pain improvement revealed that these patients had actually combined suggestions given to the CBT (e.g., regulating sleep scheduling) in addition to those received during the sleep hygiene training. Consequently, fibromyalgia patients might be expected to experience both improved sleep and better pain relief by combining suggestions for both CBT and sleep hygiene.

> **Practical pointer**
>
> Improving sleep through non-medication treatments may be linked to pain reduction.

Weight Management

Screening for and treating obesity is an essential component to fibromyalgia management. A full discussion of obesity and fibromyalgia is provided in the chapter "Obesity and Metabolic Syndrome".

Developing a Treatment Program

Because benefit has been demonstrated for several non-medication pain-relieving strategies, patients might expect to maximize their benefit by combining several effective therapies, such as exercise and cognitive-behavioral therapy. Furthermore, combining educational information about fibromyalgia and treatment outcome expectations, increased physical exercise, adaptive coping, and appropriate scheduling and pacing may help ensure better compliance with treatments. For example, patients understanding pacing limitations may be less likely to overdo exercises to provoke flares. When flares do inevitably occur, they may also approach these flares with a more productive attitude rather than catastrophizing that the treatment did not work and should be abandoned.

A meta-analysis of randomized controlled studies that included at least one educational or psychological treatment plus one exercise therapy identified significant short-term improvements in pain, fatigue, mood, quality of life, and self-efficacy ($P \leq 0.02$) [28]. Furthermore, benefits were substantially higher in studies with treatments lasting ≥ 30 h, compared with very brief interventions. Benefits realized short term, however, were lost at long-term follow-up after 6–12 months, suggesting the need for booster training to maintain improvements.

Practical pointer

Long-term benefit from non-medication treatments may be facilitated by providing periodic booster training sessions.

A recent analysis of open-label treatment with a 3-week multidisciplinary non-medication treatment program ($N = 25$) showed long-term benefits in pain reduction and aerobic fitness [29]. Patients were treated 5 h daily with educational sessions, physical exercise, CBT, and relaxation techniques. Significant improvements were noted 1 year after completing treatment for pain severity, percentage of the body affected by pain, tender point count, deep pressure pain threshold, mood, and aerobic fitness ($P < 0.001$ for each).

Summary

- Fibromyalgia patients should alternate aerobic and strengthening exercise sessions each day.
- Cognitive- and operant-behavioral therapy group treatments reduce pain by at least 50% in about half of treated patients. These benefits are maintained long term.
- Nicotine use has been linked to increased pain sensitivity, increased fibromyalgia symptoms, increased need for pain killers, and decreased analgesic potency of pain killers.
- Non-medication sleep treatments have been shown to improve sleep and, in some cases, additionally reduce pain in fibromyalgia patients.
- Combining effective non-medication techniques might maximize treatment benefit.

References

1. Bennett RM, Jones J, Turk DC, Russell IJ, Matallana L. An internet survey of 2,596 people with fibromyalgia. BMC Musculoskeletal Disorders. 2007;8:27.
2. Baranowsky J, Klose P, Musial F, et al. Qualitative systemic review of randomized controlled trials on complementary and alternative medicine treatments in fibromyalgia. Rheumatol Int. 2009;30:1–21.
3. Taylor SL, Kaur M, LoSicco K, et al. Pilot study of the effect of ultraviolet light on pain and mood in fibromyalgia syndrome. J Altern Complement Med. 2009;15:15–23.
4. Busch AJ, Barber KA, Overend TJ, Peloso PM, Schachter CL. Exercise for treating fibromyalgia syndrome. Cochrane Database Syst Rev. 2007;4:CD003786.
5. Valencia M, Alonso B, Alvarez MJ, et al. Effects of 2 physiotherapy programs on pain perception, muscular flexibility, and illness impact in women with fibromyalgia: a pilot study. J Manipulative Physiol Ther. 2009;32:84–92.
6. Langhorst J, Musial F, Klose P, Häuser W. Efficacy of hydrotherapy in fibromyalgia syndrome – a meta-analysis of randomized controlled clinical trials. Rheumatology. 2009;48:1155–9.
7. Fioravanti A, Perpignano G, Tirri G et al. Effects of mud-bath treatment on fibromyalgia patients: a randomized clinical trial. Rheumatol Int. 2007;27:1157–61.
8. Evcik D, Yigit I, Pusak H, Kavuncu V. Effectiveness of aquatic therapy in the treatment of fibromyalgia syndrome: a randomized controlled open study. Rheumatol Int. 2008;28:885–90.
9. Tsao JC. Effectiveness of massage therapy for chronic, non-malignant pain: a review. Evid Based Complement Alternat Med. 2007;4:165–79.
10. Ekici G, Bakar Y, Akbayrak T, Yuksei I. Comparison of manual lymph drainage therapy and connective tissue massage in women with fibromyalgia: a randomized controlled trial. J Manipulative Physiol Ther. 2009;32:127–33.
11. Da Silva GD, Lorenzi-Filho G, Lage LV. Effects of yoga and the addition of Tui Na in patients with fibromyalgia. J Altern Complement Med. 2007;13:1107–13.
12. Liedberg GM, Henriksson CM. Factors of importance for work disability in women with fibromyalgia: an interview study. Arthritis Rheum. 2002;47:266–74.
13. Karsdrop PA, Vlaeyen JW. Active avoidance but not activity pacing is associated with disability in fibromyalgia. Pain. 2009;147:29–35.
14. Martin-Sanchez E, Torralba E, Diaz-Domínguez E, Barriga A, Martin JL. Efficacy of acupuncture for the treatment of fibromyalgia: systematic review and meta-analysis of randomized trials. Open Rheumatol J. 2009;3:25–9.
15. Thieme K, Gracely RH. Are psychological treatments effective for fibromyalgia pain? Curr Rheumatol Rep. 2009;11:443–550.
16. Thieme K, Flor H, Turk DC. Psychological pain treatment in fibromyalgia syndrome: efficacy of operant behavioural and cognitive behavioural treatments. Arthritis Res Ther. 2006; 8:R121.
17. Thieme K, Turk DC, Flor H. Responder criteria for operant and cognitive-behavioral treatment of fibromyalgia syndrome. Arthritis Rheumat. 2007;57:830–6.
18. Menzies V, Taylor AG, Bourguignon C. Relaxation and guided imagery in Hispanic persons diagnosed with fibromyalgia: a pilot study. Fam Community Health. 2008;31:204–12.
19. Pamuk ON, Dönmez S, Cakir N. The frequency of smoking in fibromyalgia patients and its association with symptoms. Rheumatol Int. 2009;29:1311–4.
20. Pomerleau OF. Endogenous opioids and smoking – a review of progress and problems. Psychoneuroendocrinolgy. 1998;23:115–30.
21. Mansbach RS, Rovetti CC, Freeland CS. The role of monoamine neurotransmitters system in the nicotine discriminative stimulus. Drug Alcohol Depend. 1998;23:115–30.
22. Josiah DT, Vincler MA. Impact of chronic nicotine on the development and maintenance of hypersensitivity in the rat. Psychopharmacology (Berl). 2006:188:152–61.
23. John U, Hanke M, Meyer C, et al. Tobacco smoking in relation to pain in a national general population survey. Pre Med. 2006;43:477–81.

24. John U, Alte D, Hanke M, et al. Tobacco smoking in relation to analgesic drug use in a national adult population sample. Drug Alcohol Depend. 2006;85:49–55.
25. Ackerman WE, Ahmad M. Effect of cigarette smoking on serum hydrocodone levels in chronic pain patients. J Ark Med Soc. 2007;104:19–21.
26. Weingarten TN, Podduturu VR, Hooten WM, et al. Impact of tobacco use in patients presenting to a multidisciplinary outpatient treatment program for fibromyalgia. Clin J Pain. 2009;25:39–43.
27. Edinger JD, Wohlgemuth WK, Krystal AD, Rice JR. Behavioral insomnia therapy for fibromyalgia patients. A randomized clinical trial. Arch Intern Med. 2005;165:2527–35.
28. Häuser W, Bernardy K, Arnold B, Offenbächer M, Schiltenwolf M. Efficacy of multicomponent treatment in fibromyalgia syndrome: a meta-analysis of randomized controlled clinical trials. Arthritis Rheum. 2009;61:216–24.
29. Suman AL, Biagi B, Biasi G, et al. One-year efficacy of a 3-week intensive multidisciplinary non-pharmacological treatment program for fibromyalgia patients. Clin Exp Rheumatol. 2009;27:7–14.

Nutritional Supplements

Key Chapter Points

- Herbs and other supplements are used by two in five women with fibromyalgia.
- Vitamins or minerals are used by four in five fibromyalgia patients.
- Nutritional therapies that might benefit several fibromyalgia symptoms include S-adenosyl methionine, bedtime melatonin, and carnitine.
- Treatments showing modest improvements in at least one area include chlorella, vitamins C and D, coenzyme Q10, and omega-3 fatty acids.

Keywords Carnitine · Coenzyme Q10 · Fish oil · Methionine · Melatonin · Omega-3 fatty acids · Vitamin

> **Case:** Jennifer is a 34 -years old with a 7-year history of fibromyalgia. "I'll try anything to help my fibro symptoms. I've taken mega doses of vitamins and so much iron I've gotten constipated. I've heard magnesium and selenium might help, but I haven't tried them yet. Even though I'll try anything, I wish I knew what natural remedies might really help."

Utilization of herbs and other supplements is common in fibromyalgia. A survey of 434 women with fibromyalgia and 198 controls identified the use of nutritional supplements in 43% of women with fibromyalgia and 23% of controls [1]. Those with fibromyalgia reported using an average of 2.8 herbs and/or supplements per person, with 2.2 used per person by controls. The most commonly used products are shown in Table 1. Despite the higher use in women with fibromyalgia, controls were more likely to rate herbs and supplements as beneficial ($P<0.002$).

Vitamins and minerals are also commonly used. A survey of fibromyalgia patients referred to a tertiary care center reported that at least one vitamin or mineral was used by four in every five fibromyalgia patients (Table 2) [2]. The most commonly used individual vitamins and minerals were vitamins C and E and magnesium. Interestingly, a paucity of data support using these products.

D.A. Marcus, A. Deodhar, *Fibromyalgia*, DOI 10.1007/978-1-4419-1609-9_14,
© Springer Science+Business Media, LLC 2011

Table 1 Most commonly used herbs and supplements by women with fibromyalgia (based on Shaver [1])

Product	Percentage using	Median effectiveness[a]
Any herb or supplement	42.9	2
Omega essential fatty acids, fish oil, flaxseed oil	6.2	2
Glucosamine	5.3	3
Gingko	3.7	2
Garlic	3.0	1.5
Ginseng	3.0	2
Coenzyme Q10	2.8	2
Echinacea	2.5	2
Acidophilus	2.5	3
Soy	2.3	3
Primrose	2.3	3
Methylsulfonylmethane	2.3	2
Valerian	2.3	2

[a]Effectiveness was rated on a scale from 0 (not effective) to 3 (very effective)

Table 2 Vitamin and mineral usage among 289 patients with fibromyalgia referred for tertiary care (based on Wahner-Roedler [2])

Vitamin or mineral	Percentage
Any vitamin or mineral	83
Vitamin	
A	8
B-complex	25
C	35
E	31
Mega vitamin	12
Minerals	
Chromium	9
Magnesium	29
Selenium	8
Zinc	13

While fibromyalgia patients' interest in utilization of nutritional treatments is considerable, healthcare providers typically receive limited education about these products and publications commonly read by healthcare providers generally offer inadequate assessments of nutritional agents. A variety of nutritional therapies have been studied in fibromyalgia patients; however, the number of studies and use of rigorous, randomized studies is substantially less than with traditional medications or non-drug treatments like exercise and behavioral therapies. A recently published review of randomized, controlled trials of complementary or alternative medicine in fibromyalgia identified only three studies evaluating nutritional supplements: (1) a 12-week study showing significant improvement in sleep but not pain or fatigue using a product containing the anthocyanidin flavonoids (derived from cranberries, grape seeds, and bilberries), (2) a single, 6-week study showing no benefit from soy shakes, and (3) an older study published in 1991 showing significant improvements in a variety of symptoms with no reduction in tender point score with S-adenosyl methionine [3].

While the number of controlled studies testing nutritional products is limited, open-label studies have been published for a variety of nutritional treatments used to treat fibromyalgia. Although the conclusions that can be drawn from open-label studies are less strong, it is important to understand the available literature to help patients make the best choices if they decide to treat with nutritional agents. Providing suggestions for those agents most likely to be helpful may limit patients utilizing ineffective therapies. This chapter will provide a review of studies testing nutritional agents that are commonly used by fibromyalgia patients and those, like intravenous therapy, that patients are likely to read about through patient-directed, self-help resources. The strength of these recommendations should be tempered when only open-label trials are available, however, these studies can provide general guidelines for recommending treatment regimens and the types of benefits that patients might anticipate experiencing. Reviewing these data with patients may also help reinforce the need to include these treatments as part of a more comprehensive treatment program that also includes better tested and proven therapies, like exercises and behavioral treatments, rather than focusing on nutritional supplements as monotherapy.

Intravenous Nutrient Therapy

Intravenous nutrient therapy has been tested in fibromyalgia using the vitamin- and mineral-rich Myers' cocktail, which contains magnesium, calcium, hydroxocobalamin, pyridoxine, D-panthenol (vitamin B5), B-complex 100 (thiamine, riboflavin, pyridoxine, panthenol, and niacinamide), and vitamin C. A pilot study testing once weekly intravenous nutrient therapy in seven recalcitrant fibromyalgia patients for 8 weeks found improvements in pain, fatigue, energy levels, and functional ability [4].

A recent, double-blind, placebo-controlled pilot study ($N = 34$) randomized fibromyalgia patients to weekly intravenous infusions with 37 mL of Myers' cocktail or a lactated Ringer's solution placebo for 8 weeks [5]. Significant improvements occurred with both nutrient and placebo infusions, although there were no differences between improvement for patients treated with Myers' cocktail and placebo for any outcome measure (Fig. 1). Although potentially negatively impacted by the small treatment sample, this study failed to support efficacy of intravenous nutrient treatment for fibromyalgia.

Chlorella Pyrenoidosa

Fresh water alga Chlorella pyrenoidosa is rich in proteins, vitamins, and minerals. Chlorella supplementation has been tested in a small open-label ($N = 20$) [6] and a double-blind, placebo-controlled, crossover study ($N = 37$) [7]. In both studies,

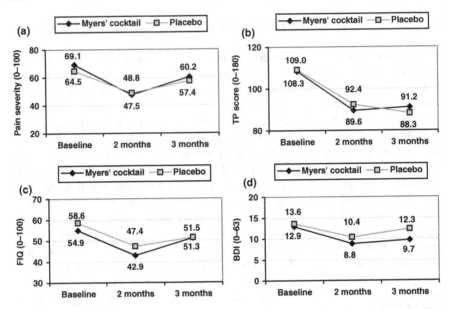

Fig. 1 Intravenous nutrient therapy (Myer's cocktail) (based on Ali [5]). (**a**) Pain severity (0 = no pain; 100 = excruciating pain). (**b**) tender point (TP) score (0 = all points are pain-free; 180 = all points are extremely tender). (**c**) Fibromyalgia Impact Questionnaire (FIQ; 0 = no negative impact; 100 = severe negative impact); an average score in the typical fibromyalgia patient = 50; scores >70 represent severe impact. (**d**) Beck Depression Inventory (BDI; 0 = no depression; 63 = severe depression). Scores >9 signify at least mild depression, with ≥16 interpreted as moderately depressed and ≥30 severely depressed

fibromyalgia patients were treated with 10 g chlorella tablet and 100 mL liquid chlorella extract daily for 2–3 months. In the open-label study, treatment was completed by 18 patients [6]. Average tender point score decreased after 2 months of treatment by 22% (*P* = 0.01). Seven patients rated their fibromyalgia symptoms as better (39%), six as unchanged (33%), and five as worse (28%). In the double-blind study, tender point severity decreased by 8% with chlorella and 2% with placebo; neither change achieved statistical significance. Functioning, however, showed greater improvement with chlorella (Fig. 2). This pair of studies highlights the importance of testing products using double-blind methodology, as the benefits achieved through double-blind trials are typically less than those seen with open-label studies, whether testing medications, nutritional, or other complementary or alternative therapies.

Practical pointer

Benefits seen in open-label studies can be exaggerated because of expectation bias. Data from more rigorous, blinded, and controlled trials usually provide a more balanced picture of outcome.

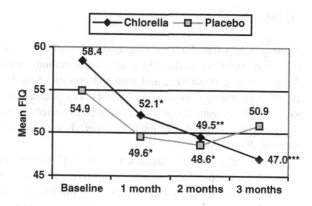

Fig. 2 Fibromyalgia Impact Questionnaire (FIQ) after treatment with chlorella vs. placebo (based on Merchant [7]). Significant change vs. baseline: $*P < 0.05$, $**P = 0.01$, $***P < 0.001$

Methionine

Essential amino acids were shown in one small study to be low in patients with fibromyalgia. In a comparison of amino acid levels in 34 fibromyalgia patients and 18 controls, patients with fibromyalgia had significantly lower plasma levels of methionine (31.6 µmol/L with fibromyalgia vs. 43.2 in controls, $P < 0.0001$), phenylalanine (62.7 µmol/L vs. 74.2 µmol/L, $P = 0.02$), threonine (67.8 µmol/L vs. 147.0 µmol/L, $P < 0.0001$), and valine (191.5 µmol/L vs. 245.6 µmol/L in controls, $P = 0.003$) [8]. The authors hypothesized that gut malabsorption defects might account for these deficits. Low methionine levels also provides a potential target for treatment with available supplements.

S-adenosyl methionine (SAMe) is primarily synthesized in the liver from dietary methionine [9]. SAMe crosses the blood–brain-barrier, where it is believed to have effects on important pain-modulating neurotransmitters, like norepinephrine, dopamine, and serotonin [9]. A review of seven clinical trials evaluating the benefit of SAMe for fibromyalgia reported statistically significant improvement in depression and a reduction in tender point count in a number of studies, although no benefits were found in the largest placebo-controlled study included in this review ($N = 44$) [9, 10]. Comparative placebo treatments were used in four studies, with a treatment comparator used in another study. Strength of the conclusions, however, is limited as these studies each included a relatively small number of patients ($N = 10$–47), withdrawals were substantial in one study (35% withdrew for unknown reasons), and additional analgesics were permitted in at least three of the studies. Based on dosing in those studies showing benefits, patients trying SAMe may consider dosing at 400 mg twice daily [9].

Practical pointer

S-adenosyl methionine (SAMe) has been studied in blinded clinical trials, although benefits have not been consistent across trials and the number of patients studied has been relatively small.

Melatonin

Although sleep disturbance is frequently co-morbid with fibromyalgia, a small study evaluating nighttime melatonin levels in nine patients with fibromyalgia, eight with chronic fatigue syndrome, and matched controls found surprisingly higher melatonin levels among fibromyalgia patients [11]. Similar melatonin levels occurred in patients with chronic fatigue syndrome and controls, with significantly higher levels among fibromyalgia patients (75.2 pg/mL with fibromyalgia vs. 58.5 pg/mL in controls, $P < 0.05$).

Interestingly, however, treatment with supplemental melatonin has been shown to be helpful in open-label treatment in fibromyalgia patients. A pilot study treating 19 fibromyalgia patients with melatonin 3 mg taken 30 min before bedtime for 4 weeks showed significant decrease in tender point count (29%, $P < 0.05$) and pain severity (33%, $P < 0.05$) [12]. (See Fig. 3.) Anecdotal data have further suggested that 6–10 mg melatonin nightly might reduce fibromyalgia pain [13].

Practical pointer

Although nocturnal melatonin deficiency has not been seen with fibromyalgia, regularly taking melatonin 30 minutes before bed improved sleep and pain in a small, open-label study.

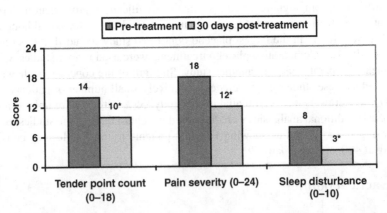

Fig. 3 Effects of 3 mg bedtime melatonin in fibromyalgia (based on Citera [12]). For each variable, a higher score represents more severe symptoms. In each case, significant improvement occurred after 1-month treatment with melatonin ($P < 0.05$)

Vitamins

Fasting vitamin levels were compared in 30 women with fibromyalgia and matched controls [14]. Concentrations of vitamins A and E were significantly lower in fibromyalgia patients (Table 3). These data support consideration for the addition of fat-soluble vitamins to patients with fibromyalgia.

Table 3 Mean vitamin levels (μmol/L) in women with fibromyalgia and matched controls (based on Akkuş [14])

Vitamin	Fibromyalgia $N = 30$	Matched controls $N = 30$	Between-group P-value
A	0.29	0.45	<0.01
C	88.00	81.75	Not significant
E	2.89	7.25	<0.001

Several studies have evaluated the benefit of vitamin supplementation for patients with fibromyalgia. The most extensive data are with vitamins C and D.

Vitamin C

A small, open-label study treated 12 women with fibromyalgia with 100 mg ascorbigen plus 400 mg broccoli powder daily for 1 month [15]. Mean physical impairment score decreased by 20% $P < 0.05$) and Fibromyalgia Impact Questionnaire Scores improved by 18% ($P < 0.05$ for both). Two weeks after discontinuing treatment, physical impairment scores reverted to near baseline.

Vitamin D

Conflicting data have been published regarding whether or not low 25-hydroxyvitamin D levels are more prevalent in patients with fibromyalgia [16–19]. Furthermore, treating patients with identified vitamin D deficiency using vitamin D supplementation failed to show pain reduction in open-label [16] and placebo-controlled [20] studies. In a recent, randomized, placebo-controlled clinical trial, patients with mild (25[OH]D 20–25 ng/mL) to moderate (25[OH]D 10–19 ng/mL) vitamin D deficiency were randomly assigned to receive 50,000 units of cholecalciferol (vitamin D_3) weekly or placebo for 8 weeks [21]. Patients with severe vitamin D deficiency (25[OH]D <10 ng/mL) were treated in an unblinded fashion. Among the initial 610 fibromyalgia patients screened for this study, 328 had sufficient vitamin D levels (54%), with mild deficiency in 119 (20%), moderate deficiency in 125 (20%), and severe deficiency in 38 (6%). Among patients randomized to vitamin D or placebo, vitamin D-treated patients experienced a modest, but significant short-term improvement in fibromyalgia assessment scores ($P = 0.03$), but no change in

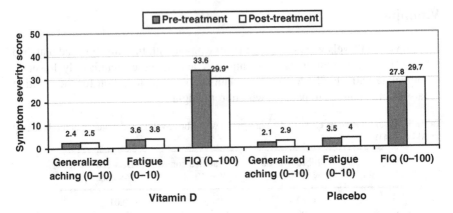

Fig. 4 Vitamin D replacement for fibromyalgia patients with vitamin D deficiency (based on Arvold [21]). FIQ = Fibromyalgia Impact Questionnaire. Possible score range is shown for each variable. For each symptoms measured, high scores represented more severe symptoms or impact. *Difference vs. pre-treatment was significant at $P = 0.03$.

pain severity or fatigue (Fig. 4). Patients with severe vitamin D deficiency showed no improvement in fibromyalgia symptoms with treatment.

Minerals

Trace minerals were studied in 32 fibromyalgia patients and 32 healthy controls [22]. Serum levels of zinc ($P = 0.001$) and magnesium ($P = 0.002$) were significantly decreased with fibromyalgia with no difference in selenium levels for both groups ($P > 0.05$). Furthermore, tender point count was correlated with serum zinc level ($P = 0.008$), while magnesium was linked to fatigue ($P = 0.003$). Although studies have not directly tested benefit from mineral replacement, these data suggest that such replacement might possibly be beneficial.

Coenzyme Q10

Coenzyme Q10 is essential for aerobic metabolism, with antioxidant properties that protect cells from the damaging effects of reactive oxygen species (harmful molecules formed by incomplete reduction of oxygen, e.g., free radicals and peroxides). A study comparing plasma samples from 40 fibromyalgia patients and 30 controls found antioxidant coenzyme Q10 levels to be twice as high in fibromyalgia patients compared with controls (355.8 nM/L vs. 174.4 nM/L, $P < 0.001$) [23]. Despite higher levels in plasma, concentrations in mononuclear cells were 40% lower in fibromyalgia patients (138.4 pmol/mg protein vs. 225.1 pmol/mg protein, $P < 0.01$). Furthermore, fibromyalgia mononuclear cells showed significantly higher production of reactive oxygen species (16.8 au vs. 10.4 au, $P = 0.025$). Incubating fibromyalgia cells with supplemental coenzyme Q10 significantly reduced the production of reactive oxygen species to 11.9 au ($P = 0.03$). These data support that coenzyme Q10 supplementation might be beneficial for fibromyalgia patients for reducing the effects of oxidative stress, although clinical benefits were not evaluated.

A small, open-label study tested clinical benefits of coenzyme Q10 and Ginkgo biloba in 23 patients with fibromyalgia [24]. Subjects took two coenzyme Q10 100 mg capsules and two Ginkgo biloba 100 mg tablets daily for 3 months. Outcome was measured using the validated, Dartmouth Primary Care Cooperative Information Project/World Organization of Family Doctors (COOP/WONCA) Questionnaire. This questionnaire scores six domains (physical fitness, emotional problems, daily activities, social activities, change in health, general health perception, and pain) from 1 to 5, with total scores ranging from a best quality of life of 5 to worst quality of life of 35. After 3 months of treatment, average quality of life scores improved significantly by 16% ($P < 0.02$) and two in three patients rated themselves as better (Fig. 5). As a comparison, a recent assessment of fibromyalgia patients using the COOP/WONCA showed a similar average COOP/WONCA quality of life score of 28.1 [25].

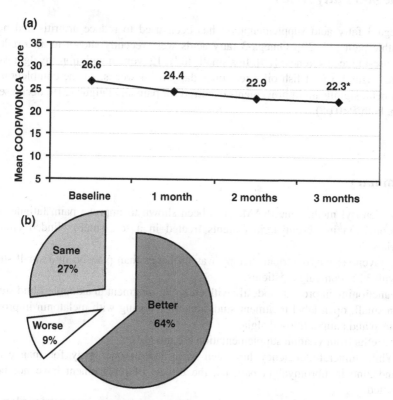

Fig. 5 Open-label coenzyme Q10 plus Ginkgo biloba in fibromyalgia (based on Lister [24]). (a) Quality of life. Change vs. baseline was significant: *$P < 0.02$. (b) Patient self-rating of how he/she felt at the end at 3 months

Carnitine

Early research in fibromyalgia inconsistently showed carnitine deficiency in some patients with fibromyalgia [26]. In a double-blind clinical trial, 102 fibromyalgia patients were randomized to treatment with acetyl L-carnitine or placebo for 10 weeks [26]. Patients were treated with one intramuscular injection of acetyl L-carnitine 500 mg or placebo followed by two capsules of acetyl L-carnitine 500 mg or placebo daily for 2 weeks. After 2 weeks, patients in both groups took three capsules of carnitine or placebo daily for the remaining 8 weeks. Although initial improvement in pain threshold and tender point count was similar for patients supplemented with carnitine vs. placebo, significantly better improvement was noted after 10 weeks with carnitine. After 10 weeks, improvement in musculoskeletal pain and depression were also significantly better with carnitine.

Omega-3 Fatty Acids

Omega-3 fatty acid supplementation has been used to reduce arthritis and neuropathic pain [27, 28]. Omega-3 fatty acids were recently shown to also reduce exercise-induced soreness [29]. In a small study, 12 women with fibromyalgia were treated with 1.5 g of fish oil three times daily for 4 weeks. At the completion of treatment, significant improvements occurred for pain and fatigue (21% decrease in each, both $P<0.05$).

Summary

- S-adenosyl methionine (SAMe) has been shown to improve pain, fatigue, and depression in fibromyalgia patients treated in a few small, blinded clinical trials.
- Intravenous micronutrient therapy was no better than placebo in a small study with 34 fibromyalgia patients.
- Functioning improved modestly with chlorella treatment in a double-blind study.
- In small, open-label treatment study, bedtime dosing with melatonin improved sleep and pain in fibromyalgia.
- Benefits from vitamin supplementation are modest.
- While mineral deficiency has been identified in one study for magnesium and zinc in fibromyalgia patients, the effects of replacement have not been tested.
- Although short-term treatment with carnitine produces similar results to placebo, carnitine shows superior improvements in pain and mood after 10 weeks of treatment.

References

1. Shaver JL, Wilbur J, Lee, H, Robinson FP, Wang E. Self-reported medication and herb/supplement use by women with and without fibromyalgia. J Women's Health. 2009;18:709–16.

2. Wahner-Roedler DL, Elkin PL, Vincent A, et al. Use of complementary and alternative medical therapies by patients referred to a fibromyalgia treatment program at a tertiary care center. Mayo Clin Proc. 2005;80:55–60.

3. De Silva V, El-Metwally A, Ernst E, Lewith G, Macfarlane GJ. Evidence for the efficacy of complementary and alternative medicines in the management of fibromyalgia: a systematic review. Rheumatology. 2010;49:1063–8.

4. Massey PB. Reduction of fibromyalgia symptoms through intravenous nutrient therapy: results of a pilot clinical trial. Altern Ther Health Med. 2007;13:32–4.

5. Ali A, Njike VY, Northrup V, et al. Intravenous micronutrient therapy (Myers; Cocktail) for fibromyalgia: a placebo-controlled pilot study. J Altern Complement Med. 2009;15:247–57.

6. Merchant RE, Carmack CA, Wise CM. Nutritional supplementation with Chlorella pyrenoidosa for patients with fibromyalgia syndrome: a pilot study. Phytother Res. 2000;14:167–73.

7. Merchant RE, Andre CA. A review of recent clinical trials of the nutritional supplement Chlorella pyrenoidosa in the treatment of fibromyalgia, hypertension, and ulcerative colitis. Altern Ther Health Med. 2001;7:79–91.

8. Bazzichi L, Palego L, Giannaccini G, et al. Altered amino acid homeostasis in subjects affected by fibromyalgia. Clin Biochem. 2009;42:1064–70.

9. Fetrow CW, Avila JR. Efficacy of the dietary supplement S-adenosyl-L-methionine. Ann Pharmacother. 2001;35:1414–25.

10. Sarac AJ, Gur A. Complementary and alternative medical therapies in fibromyalgia. Curr Pharm Des. 2006;12:47–57.

11. Korszun Am Sackett-Lundeen L, Papadopoulos E, et al. Melatonin levels in women with fibromyalgia and chronic fatigue syndrome. J Rheumatol. 1999;26:2675–80.

12. Citera G, Arias MA, Maldonado-Cocco JA, et al. The effect of melatonin in patients with fibromyalgia: a pilot study. Clin Rheumatol. 2000;19:9–13.

13. Reiter RJ, Acuna-Castroviejo D, Tan DX. Melatonin therapy in fibromyalgia. Curr Pain Headache Rep. 2007;11:339–42.

14. Akkuş S, Naziroğlu M, Eriş S, Yalman K, Yilmaz N, Yener M. Levels of lipid peroxidation, nitric oxide, and antioxidant vitamins in plasma of patients with fibromyalgia. Cell Biochem Funct. 2009;27:181–5.

15. Bramwell B, Ferguson S, Scarlett N, Macintosh A. The use of ascorbigen in the treatment of fibromyalgia patients: a preliminary trial. Altern Med Rev. 2000;5:455–62.

16. Block SR. Vitamin D deficiency is not associated with nonspecific musculoskeletal pain syndromes including fibromyalgia. Mayo Clin Proc. 2004;79:1585–6.

17. Huisman AM, White KP, Algra A, et al. Vitamin D levels in women with systemic lupus erythematosus and fibromyalgia. J Rheumatol. 2001;28:2535–9.

18. Plotmikoff GA, Quigley JM. Prevalence of severe hypovitaminosis D in patients with persistent, nonspecific musculoskeletal pain. Mayo Clin Proc. 2003;78:1463–70.

19. Tandeter H, Grynbaum M, Zuili I, Shany S, Shvartzman P. Serum 25-OH vitamin D levels in patients with fibromyalgia. Isr Med Assoc J. 2009;11:399–42.

20. Warner AE, Arnspiger SA. Diffuse musculoskeletal pain is not associated with low vitamin D levels or improved by treatment with vitamin D. J Clin Rheumatol. 2008;14:12–6.

21. Arvold DS, Odean MJ, Dornfeld MP, et al. Correlation of symptoms with vitamin D deficiency and symptom response to cholecalciferol treatment: a randomized controlled trial. Endrocr Pract. 2009;15:203–12.

22. Sendur OF, Tastaban E, Turan Y, Ulman C. The relationship between serum trace element levels and clinical parameters in patients with fibromyalgia. Rheumatol Int. 2008;28:1117–21.

23. Cordero MD, Moreno-Fernández AM, deMiguel M, et al. Coenzyme Q10 distribution in blood is altered in patients with fibromyalgia. Clin Biochem. 2009;42:732–35.
24. Lister RE. An open, pilot study to evaluate the potential benefits of coenzyme Q10 combined with Ginkgo biloba extract in fibromyalgia syndrome. J Int Med Res. 2002;30:195–9.
25. Peña ME, Garcia RJ, Olalla JM, et al. Impact of the most frequent chronic health conditions on the quality of life among people aged >15 years in Madrid. Eur J Public Health. 2010;20: 78–84.
26. Rossini M, Di Munno O, Valentini G, et al. Double-blind, multicenter trial comparing acetyl l-carnitine with placebo in the treatment of fibromyalgia patients. Clin Exp Rheumatol. 2007;25:182–8.
27. Fetterman JW, Zdanowicz MM. Therapeutic potential of n-3 polyunsaturated fatty acids in disease. Am J Health Syst Pharm. 2009;66:1169–79.
28. Ko GD, Nowacki NB, Arseneau L, Eitel M, Hum A. Omega-3 Fatty acids for neuropathic pain: case series. Clin J Pain. 2010;26:168–72.
29. Tartibain B, Maleki BH, Abbasi A. The effects of ingestion of omega-3 fatty acids on perceived pain and external symptoms of delayed onset muscle soreness in untrained men. Clin J Sport Med. 2009;19:115–9.

Clinical Handouts

Key Chapter Points

- Charting tools can effectively identify and record patient disability and psychological distress.
- Charting tools can help clearly measure patient response to treatment.
- Patient educational handouts can help supplement messages given by healthcare providers.
- Patient handouts can teach patients the basics of exercises, relaxation, and other pain-relieving therapies.

Keywords Drug · Exercise · Fibromyalgia · Relaxation · Supplement

Patient education, training, treatment adherence, and progress can be facilitated by utilizing standardized written tools. This chapter includes both charting tools to assist with patient evaluation and monitor treatment progress, and patient educational handouts to reinforce helpful self-management pain-relieving therapies. The tools are designed to augment rather than replace clinical interactions. Sending patients home with handouts can help support messages relayed during your visit and also serve as motivational tools to remind patients to regularly perform important pain management therapies. Patient progress may be monitored through review of patient diary logs and utilization of charting assessment tools that can readily record treatment benefits over time. These resources are available for download through the publisher's Web site at http://extras.springer.com/.

Charting Assessment and Treatment Documentation Forms

1. Fibromyalgia tender point examination
2. Fibromyalgia patient assessment recording sheet
3. Revised Fibromyalgia Impact Questionnaire
4. Screening for psychological distress
5. Screen for locus of control

D.A. Marcus, A. Deodhar, *Fibromyalgia*, DOI 10.1007/978-1-4419-1609-9_15,
© Springer Science+Business Media, LLC 2011

Charting documentation form 1. Fibromyalgia tender point examination (Reprinted from Marcus DA. Chronic Pain. A Primary Care Guide to Practical Management. Totowa, NJ: Humana Press, 2005.)

Name:_____   Date:_____/_____/_____

- Test each labeled spot by exerting 4 kg of pressure with the thumb (watch for the nail bed to blanch).
- Record pain severity at each spot in the circles from 0 (none) to 10 (excruciating).
- Calculate and log tender point count (number of painful tender points scored >0) and tender point score (sum of all recorded scores).
    - Tender point count: _____
    - Tender point score: _____

Charting documentation form 2. Fibromyalgia patient assessment recording sheet

Use this chart to follow your patient's progress and treatment response for common, treatable fibromyalgia symptoms.

Name:_____

Fibromyalgia symptom	Visit log (Record visit dates in columns below)				
	Initial visit	Follow-up	Follow-up	Follow-up	Follow-up
Tender point count (range=0–18)					
Tender point score (range=0–180)					
Average pain severity (0=no pain, 10=excruciating and disabling pain)					
Average number of hours of nighttime sleep (healthy sleep in adults=7–9 h nightly)					
Sleep Quality Scale over last 24 h (0=best sleep, 10=worst sleep)					
Check the visit box for each of the following symptoms that is problematic. Add notations to each box to expand, if helpful					
Disability for work or household chores					
Disability for leisure, family, or social activities					
Sleep disturbance					
Bowel problems					
Troublesome headaches					
Excess weight					
Depression or anxiety					

Charting documentation form 3. Revised Fibromyalgia Impact Questionnaire [FIQR]
(Adapted from Bennett [1])

Name:_____   Date:_____/_____/_____

Question 1. Circle how difficult it has been to do each of the following tasks over the
past week from 0 (no difficulty) to 10 (very difficult):

Brush or comb your hair	0 1 2 3 4 5 6 7 8 9 10
Walk continuously for 20 min	0 1 2 3 4 5 6 7 8 9 10
Prepare a homemade meal	0 1 2 3 4 5 6 7 8 9 10
Vacuum, scrub, or sweep floors	0 1 2 3 4 5 6 7 8 9 10
Lift and carry a full bag of groceries	0 1 2 3 4 5 6 7 8 9 10
Climb one flight of stairs	0 1 2 3 4 5 6 7 8 9 10
Change bedding	0 1 2 3 4 5 6 7 8 9 10
Sit in a chair for 45 min	0 1 2 3 4 5 6 7 8 9 10
Shop for groceries	0 1 2 3 4 5 6 7 8 9 10

Question 2. Rate the overall impact fibromyalgia has had over the last week from 0
(never) to 10 (always):

Fibromyalgia prevented me from
accomplishing what I wanted to this week   0 1 2 3 4 5 6 7 8 9 10

I was completely overwhelmed by
fibromyalgia this week   0 1 2 3 4 5 6 7 8 9 10

Question 3. Rate the intensity of these fibromyalgia symptoms over the past week
from 0 (none) to 10 (very severe)

Pain	0 1 2 3 4 5 6 7 8 9 10
Stiffness	0 1 2 3 4 5 6 7 8 9 10
Depression	0 1 2 3 4 5 6 7 8 9 10
Anxiety	0 1 2 3 4 5 6 7 8 9 10
Tenderness to touch	0 1 2 3 4 5 6 7 8 9 10
Balance problems	0 1 2 3 4 5 6 7 8 9 10
Sensitivity to loud noise, bright lights, odors, and cold	0 1 2 3 4 5 6 7 8 9 10

Question 4. Rate the following over the past week from 0 (not a problem) to 10 (very
severe problem)

Energy level	0 1 2 3 4 5 6 7 8 9 10
Sleep quality	0 1 2 3 4 5 6 7 8 9 10
Memory	0 1 2 3 4 5 6 7 8 9 10

Scoring the FIQR:
1. Add each selected rating for all items in Question 1 and divide by 3.
2. Add ratings for both items in Question 2.
3. Add ratings for all items in Questions 3 and 4; divide total by 2.
4. Add these three scores together for the total FIQR score. Maximum total score =
   100. Average score in fibromyalgia patients = 50. Scores >70 represent severe
   impact.

Charting documentation form 4. Screening for psychological distress

A. Depression screening (Adapted from Hilton and colleagues' Depression in Medically Ill screen or DMI-10 [2]. Reprinted from Marcus DA. Chronic Pain. A Primary Care Guide to Practical Management. Totowa, NJ: Humana Press, 2009.)

Name:_____   Date:_____/_____/_____

Please rate each statement, considering how you have been feeling in the last 2–3 days compared with how you normally feel:

	Not true Score=0	Slightly true Score=1	Moderately true Score=2	Very true Score=3
I find myself stewing over things.				
I feel more vulnerable than usual.				
I am critical of or hard on myself.				
I feel guilty				
Nothing seems to cheer me up.				
I feel like I've lost my core or essence.				
I feel depressed.				
I feel less worthwhile.				
I feel hopeless or helpless.				
I feel distant from other people.				

Scoring: Sum scores from each question. A total score ≥ 9 suggests depression.

B. Anxiety screening (adapted from Spitzer and colleagues' General Anxiety Disorder-7 (GAD-7) [3]. Reprinted from Marcus DA. Chronic Pain. A Primary Care Guide to Practical Management. Totowa, NJ: Humana Press, 2009.)

Name:_____   Date:_____/_____/_____

Choose the one description for each item that best describes **how many days** have you have been bothered by each of the following over the past **2 weeks**:

	None Score=0	Several Score=1	7 or more Score=2	Nearly every day Score=3
Feeling nervous, anxious, or on edge				
Unable to stop worrying				
Worrying too much about different things				
Problems relaxing				
Feeling restless or unable to sit still				
Feeling irritable or easily annoyed				
Being afraid that something awful might happen				

Scoring: Sum scores from each question. A total score 5–9 suggests mild anxiety, while a score ≥10 suggests moderate–severe anxiety.

Charting documentation form 5. Screen for locus of control (adapted from Wallston et al. [4, 5])

Name:_____ Date:_____/_____/_____

	Disagree			Agree		
Statements	**Strongly**	**Moderately**	**Slightly**	**Strongly**	**Moderately**	**Slightly**
1. If my fibromyalgia worsens, my own behavior will determine how soon I will feel better						
2. With my fibromyalgia, what will be will be						
3. If I see the doctor regularly, I am less likely to have problems with fibromyalgia						
4. Most things that affect my fibromyalgia happen by chance						
5. Whenever my fibromyalgia worsens, I should consult a medically trained professional						
6. I am directly responsible for my fibromyalgia getting better or worse						
7. Other people play a big role in whether my fibromyalgia improves, stays the same, or gets worse						
8. Whatever goes wrong with my fibromyalgia is my own fault						
9. Luck plays a big part in determining how my fibromyalgia improves						
10. In order for my fibromyalgia to improve, it is up to other people to see that the right things happen						
11. Whatever improvement occurs with my fibromyalgia is largely a matter of good fortune						
12. The main thing that affects my fibromyalgia is what I do myself						
13. I deserve credit when my fibromyalgia improves and blame when it worsens						
14. Following doctor's orders to the letter is the best way to keep my fibromyalgia from getting worse						
15. It's a matter of fate if my fibromyalgia worsens						
16. If I am lucky, my fibromyalgia will get better						
17. If my fibromyalgia worsens, it is because I have not been taking proper care of myself						
18. The type of help I get from others determines how soon my fibromyalgia will improve						

Choose whether you agree or disagree with each statement and rate how strongly you agree or disagree.

Scoring locus of control:
Assign the following numeric values to the ratings above:
- Strongly disagree = 1
- Moderately disagree = 2
- Slightly disagree = 3
- Slightly agree = 4
- Moderately agree = 5
- Strongly agree = 6

To determine the score for **Internal Locus of Control**, add scores for questions:
    1, 6, 8, 12, 13, and 17

To determine the score for **Powerful Others Locus of Control**, add scores for questions:
    3, 5, 7, 10, 14, and 18

To determine the score for **Chance Locus of Control**, add scores for questions:
    2, 4, 9, 11, 15, and 16

Possible score range for each locus = 6–36. A higher score represents a greater placement of locus of control in that category.

Patient Educational Handouts

1. Understanding fibromyalgia
2. Whole body stretches for fibromyalgia
3. Exercise for fibromyalgia
4. Pain management techniques
5. Relaxation techniques
6. Sleep management for fibromyalgia patients
7. Nutritional supplements for fibromyalgia

Patient Handout 1: Understanding Fibromyalgia

What is Fibromyalgia?

Fibromyalgia is a condition causing increased sensitivity to pain. Fibromyalgia causes widespread body pain, as well as other problems like fatigue, poor sleep, numbness, bowel and bladder problems, depression, and anxiety. Fortunately, fibromyalgia symptoms do *not* progress to cause severe weakness, paralysis, or the inability to move or walk.

If you have fibromyalgia, you will probably hear that your physical examination and tests are normal. Most tests your doctor can do are designed to look for major problems in the nerves, muscles, and joints. You can still have disabling pain and other symptoms caused by fibromyalgia when the tests for these problems are normal.

Why Do I have Fibromyalgia?

If you have fibromyalgia – you are not alone. About 2–3% of all adults have fibromyalgia. Women are affected three times more often than men. Some people get fibromyalgia after an illness or trauma, while it seems to start out of the blue for others. Researchers have identified changes in nerve and muscle physiology, hormones, inflammation, and genetic factors in people with fibromyalgia. Although doctors still have not figured out exactly what is causing fibromyalgia, studies do show that the symptoms are very real and caused by real, biological changes in your body. Often these changes will not be detected with the usual testing that can be done at the doctor's office.

How Is Fibromyalgia Treated?

The good news is that there are lots of effective treatments that help reduce fibromyalgia symptoms. About half of those patients with fibromyalgia will report that their symptoms are much or very much better after a couple of years. So there is a light at the end of the tunnel – you just have to be patient while you get there.

Most people need to use non-medication treatments, such as:

- Aerobic exercise 20 minutes daily for 2 or 3 days each week
- Strengthening exercises 2 or 3 days each week
- Psychological pain management techniques, like relaxation therapy, cognitive-behavioral therapy, operant-behavioral therapy, and stress management

Some patients also use medications. While no medications were specifically designed to treat fibromyalgia, several drugs used for other health problems have also been found to help fibromyalgia:

- Mood elevators, like duloxetine [Cymbalta] and milnacipran [Savella]
- Seizure drugs, like pregabalin [Lyrica]
- Sleep drugs, like sodium oxybate [Xyrem]

Each of these drugs has been shown to reduce a wide range of fibromyalgia symptoms, including pain, disability, depression, and sleep problems. Most pain killers are not very helpful for fibromyalgia.

Where Can I Learn More?

Good information about the diagnosis and treatment of fibromyalgia can be found at these Web sites:

- http://familydoctor.org
- http://fmaware.org
- http://fmpartnership.org
- http://www.hopkins-arthritis.org
- http://www.myalgia.com

Patient Handout 2: Whole Body Stretches for Fibromyalgia

Stretching exercises are an important way to help prepare your muscles and joints for your aerobic exercise. Stretches can also help you wind down at the end of the day before going to bed. You may want to try these stretches after first warming your muscles in a warm shower.

Perform each stretch slowly. Only stretch until you first feel a stretching sensation. Then hold the stretch for 5 seconds, relax, and repeat 3–10 times. Try doing these stretches while you listen to music.

If your pain levels are consistently increased after stretching, reduce the extent of the stretch and review your exercise program with your physical therapist.

Starting Position

Lie flat on the floor. If you feel uncomfortable flat on your back, bend your knees, and press the small of your back into the floor.

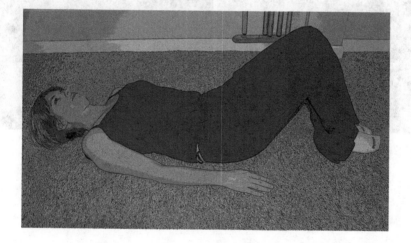

Neck Rotation

Start with your head looking up at the ceiling. Then rotate your neck slowly to the left. Try to place your left ear flat on the floor. Hold for 5 seconds. Return to center and relax. Then rotate to the right and hold for 5 seconds. Return to center and relax.

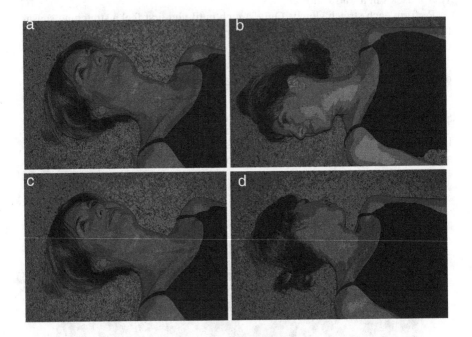

Shoulder Rollover

Hold each arm out at the shoulder so your body makes a giant cross. Keeping your arms on the floor, bend your elbows to make a 90° angle, keeping your arms flat on the floor. This is your starting position. Keep your arms on the floor between the shoulder and the elbow and rotate your forearms up and over. Then rotate back to the starting position.

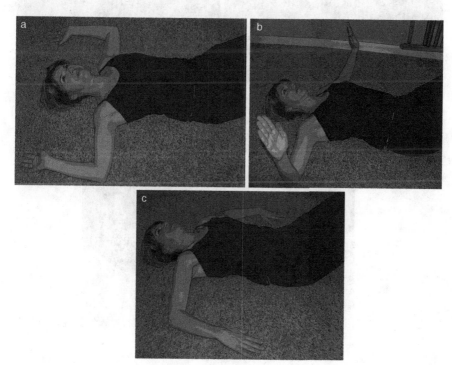

Shoulder Stick 'em up

Take a deep breath and raise your arms over your head, like someone said, "Stick 'em up!" Breathe out and reach around with your arms in a half circle, first up toward the ceiling, then down to your sides. Breathe in and reach overhead again.

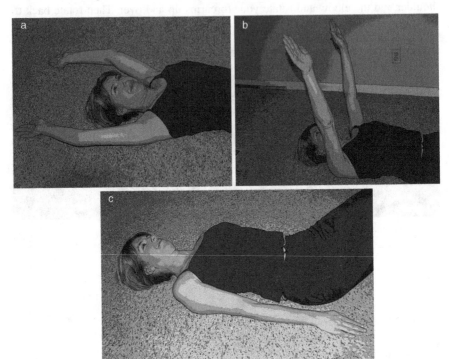

Upper Body Twist

Lift your left arm toward the ceiling and grab your left wrist with your right hand. Keeping your left arm straight (do not bend your left elbow), pull your left arm across your chest to the right. Then turn chin to the left. Hold. Repeat with the right arm.

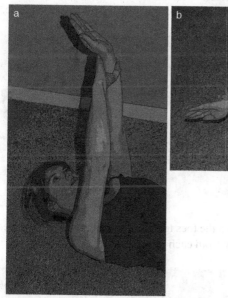
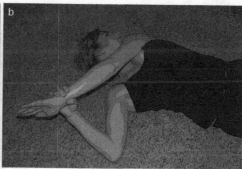

Reach Away

Stretch your left arm over your head and point your right toe. Stretch your arm and leg away from each other. Hold. Repeat with the right arm and left leg.

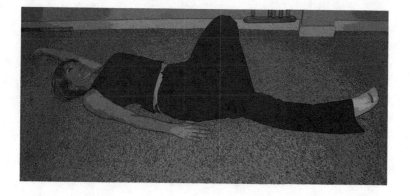

Pelvis Twist

Make sure you begin this stretch with your knees bent and the small of your back pressed into the floor. Throughout this stretch, keep your knees together and your shoulders touching the floor. Slowly lower your knees to the floor at the right, causing a rotation of your pelvis. Turn your head to the left, away from your knees. Hold. Return knees and head to the center. Then lower your knees to the left and look right. Keep your head and shoulders on the floor to allow your pelvis to rotate.

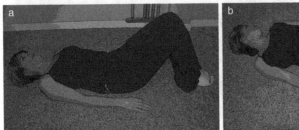
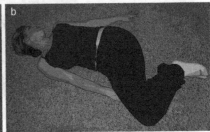

Happy Feet

Spread your feet about 2 feet apart. Turn the toes together in the middle. Hold. Then turn both feet so your toes are far away from each other. Hold.

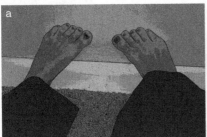
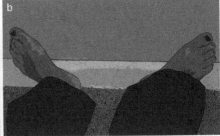

Patient Handout 3: Exercise for Fibromyalgia

Exercise has been proven to be one of the most helpful treatments for reducing fibromyalgia symptoms. The most effective exercises for fibromyalgia patients include:

- **Aerobic exercise**
    - Do whole body stretches before beginning your workout
    - After a 5-minute warm-up, exercise for a total of 20 minutes, followed by a 5-minute cooldown
    - Do aerobic exercise at least 3 days each week
    - Doing aerobic exercise in warm water may be beneficial

- **Strength training**
    - Work up to doing 8–12 repetitions per strength exercise
    - Do strength training 2–3 days per week

Keeping track of your exercise progress in daily diaries can help motivate you to stick with your program. You should also share these logs with your healthcare provider to help assess your program and its benefits.

Talk to your doctor before starting any exercise program to help determine what is best for you. Good aerobic exercise can include:

- Walking in the mall, on hiking trails, or on a school track
- Biking
- Swimming

When you start any new aerobic program, begin slowly and increase the intensity about every 4–5 days. If your pain worsens, temporarily reduce your activity to the level that you previously tolerated for about 2–3 days, then try increasing again.

Exercise Logs

Check the box that corresponds to your level of exercise each day. Target doing at least 20 minutes of aerobic exercise at least 3 days each week. Watch to see that you do not miss too many exercise days and that you GRADUALLY increase your level of exercise. You should also try to do strength training 2–3 days each week. You can use small weights at the gym or from your sporting goods store or use small soup or fruit cans for hand weights. More repetitions with smaller weights will be more beneficial than doing only a couple repetitions with heavier weights.

Weekly walking log:

	Sunday	Monday	Tuesday	Wednesday	Thursday	Friday	Saturday
1 mile							
$\frac{1}{2}$ mile							
$\frac{1}{4}$ mile							
$\frac{1}{8}$ mile							
Strength training							

Weekly biking or swimming log:

	Sunday	Monday	Tuesday	Wednesday	Thursday	Friday	Saturday
20 minutes							
15 minutes							
10 minutes							
5 minutes							
Strength training							

Patient Handout 4: Pain Management Techniques

Two pain management techniques that have been proven to reduce fibromyalgia symptoms are *cognitive-behavioral therapy* and *operant-behavioral therapy*. Many times, working with a behavioral psychologist is helpful to master these skills.

Cognitive-behavioral therapy involves changing how you *think* about your pain. Change your thoughts from negative to positive. Negative thoughts about fibromyalgia include catastrophic thinking that the pain will never improve, that nothing you do will ever help, and that achieving pain relief is hopeless. Typical negative thoughts might be:

- "I'll never get better!"
- "It's hopeless."
- "I'm doomed to spend the day on the couch."
- "Nothing I do every makes a difference."

Talk to yourself with positive messages.

- "I'm taking control of my fibromyalgia 1 day at a time."
- "If I take a break and practice some pain techniques, my pain level should become more manageable."
- "Next time, I'll need to schedule my activities better so I don't try to do too much and get so wiped out."
- "Sticking with my exercise program will help reduce my disability."

Set realistic goals. Do not expect your treatment to cure your fibromyalgia. Here are some realistic goals:

- Decrease pain severity from severe to moderate
- Decrease the time you spend in bed or lying on the sofa
- Increase your ability to do household chores and attend family activities or social functions
- Reduce problems with your mood or anxiety
- Improve your sleep
- Improve your bowel habits
- Reliance on medications

Try setting specific goals for yourself. Instead of "wanting to be more active," set targets like "being able to shop for 20 minutes," "being able to walk 20 minutes each day," and "being able to cook dinner for the family."

Schedule your tasks for success. If you can break tasks into smaller segments, you will have great success. For example, if you want to do the laundry, first load and run the machine in the morning, then do your stretching exercises and a 10-minutes walk. Switch clothes to the dryer in the afternoon and practice some deep breathing.

Finally, fold the clothes while sitting down watching television in the evening. If you break tasks down and take breaks between segments, you will have better success.

Operant-behavioral therapy involves changing how you *act* with your pain. When we have pain, we often talk about our pain, moan, grimace, or move our bodies differently. When other people see and hear us doing this, they will probably respond to our pain behaviors. Sometimes these responses can encourage you to do things that will not really help your symptoms. For example, some people may talk with you about how bad pain is or they may encourage you to take extra pain pills, go to bed, or call the doctor. People may also add to our negative thinking by saying things like, "Your fibromyalgia always interferes with our fun" or "Every time we try to do something, your fibromyalgia gets in the way." When other people react this way, it can encourage you to do things that are not helpful for your fibromyalgia.

Operant-behavioral therapy trains you to try not to display so many pain behaviors.

- Pay attention to how much you talk about your pain with others and try to shift conversations to more positive topics.
- Watch how you move and walk when your symptoms are bothering you and try to move normally.
- Catch yourself when you hear yourself moaning or groaning as you move.

Operant-behavioral therapy also trains the people usually around you to respond to your pain by encouraging you to do the things your doctor has recommended for your fibromyalgia.

- Tell family and friends, "Let's not talk about my pain. What's new with you?"
- Let family and friends know that you would like them to encourage you to stay active by suggesting activities that help keep you moving.
- Remind family and friends that you want to keep up with your chores and not to jump in to finish them for you if you take longer than usual.
- Family and friends can suggest fun activities to help distract you from your symptoms.

Patient Handout 5: Relaxation Techniques

Relaxation techniques can help reduce pain levels and are most helpful when combined with other pain management techniques, like cognitive-behavioral therapy. Two effective types of relaxation are *progressive muscle relaxation* and *cue-controlled relaxation*. Many times, working with a behavioral psychologist is helpful to master these skills.

Sit in a comfortable chair in a quiet room. Do not cross your arms or legs and make sure your feet are resting flat on the floor. Close your eyes and begin the exercises listed below. When you are first learning these techniques, practice them once or twice a day for about 15 or 20 minutes. Try to practice when your symptoms are milder. Once you have regularly practiced and mastered these techniques, you will be able to use them whenever you feel yourself starting to tense, in anticipation of stress, or when your fibromyalgia symptoms start to get more severe.

Progressive muscle relaxation involves contracting and then relaxing muscles throughout your body.

- Close your eyes.
- Practice tensing and then relaxing individual muscles in different parts of your body. Start with the muscles in your feet and move through the muscle groups up to your face.
- As you tense each muscle, hold the tension for 10–15 seconds, and then release it.
- Tense and release the muscles in your legs, then abdomen, then arms, then shoulders, then neck, then jaw, then eyes, then forehead.
- Focus on how the muscles feel when they are no longer tensed.
- When you have practiced this exercise a number of times, you will begin to recognize when your muscles first start to get tense. As you feel your muscles tense, take a few minutes and practice progressive muscle relaxation to help relax them.

Cue-controlled relaxation involves deep breathing while repeating the word "relax."

- Take a slow, deep, abdominal breath.
- To make sure you are doing an abdominal breath, place your hand over your belly when you breathe. Feel your belly move in and out with each deep breath.
- After breathing in, hold your breath for 5–10 seconds. Then slowly exhale and repeat the word "relax" as you blow out air. Repeat.
- When you have practiced this exercise a number of times, try closing your eyes and taking deep abdominal breaths before dealing with stressful situations. You can try this when standing in the shower while waiting in line at the store, before talking to your teenager or spouse, or before meeting with your boss or your child's teacher. You can also use cue-controlled relaxation when you start to feel stressed or your fibromyalgia symptoms worsen.

Patient Handout 6: Sleep Management for Fibromyalgia Patients

Getting adequate sleep is important for good health. Poor sleep increases your risk for becoming obese and developing diabetes because sleep helps curb your appetite and control your body's metabolism of glucose. People with poor sleep also have higher levels of inflammation chemicals that can increase your risk for high blood pressure and heart disease. Interestingly, sleep is also linked to pain sensitivity. People with poor sleep actually have a lower pain threshold, so your pain will be more severe when you are sleeping poorly.

How much sleep do I need? Adults typically need 7–9 hours of sleep each night for good health. Unfortunately, about four in every five patients with fibromyalgia will have problems with sleep. Getting better sleep will help make your other pain treatments work better.

Talk to your doctor about your sleep. Make sure you let your doctor know what sleep problems you may be having. A good way to rate your sleep is to use the *Sleep Quality Scale*:

> *Rate your sleep quality over the last 24 hours*
> *0 = best possible sleep   10 = worst possible sleep*

Your doctor can suggest a variety of changes that may improve your sleep. Occasionally, patients need medications to help regulate sleep. Talk to your doctor about medications that have also been shown to reduce other fibromyalgia symptoms:

- Antidepressants duloxetine [Cymbalta], milnacipran [Savella], and amitriptyline [Elavil]
- Antiepileptic drugs pregabalin [Lyrica] and gabapentin [Neurotin]
- Sleep disorder drug sodium oxybate [Xyrem]

Practice These Good Sleep Habits

- Daily habits to help with sleep

  - Avoid excessive daytime napping. Do not nap more than once each afternoon or for longer than 45 minutes.
  - Do aerobic exercise daily

- Be prepared for bed

  - Reduce evening stimulants, like caffeine and nicotine
  - Do not drink alcohol before going to bed
  - Practice relaxation techniques at bedtime
  - Avoid stimulating activities during the couple of hours before bed
  - Dim ambient room lighting 1–2 hours before bed to prepare for sleep

- Add a light evening snack before bed, like a bowl of cereal or glass of milk
- Make sure your bedroom is pleasantly cool

- Bedtime habits

  - Establish and maintain regular sleep and rise times
  - Use bed only for sleep and sex
  - Go to bed only when sleepy
  - Do not watch television or read in bed
  - If too much ambient light enters the bedroom, invest in an eye mask
  - If noises in the bedroom prevent sleep, try using ear plugs
  - If you are unable to fall asleep after 15 minutes, get up and go to another room. Only return to bed when you are sleepy.

Patient Handout 7: Nutritional Supplements for Fibromyalgia

You might be able to use nutritional supplements to help reduce some of your fibromyalgia symptoms. People with fibromyalgia are twice as likely to use vitamins, minerals, and herbs as other people. If you would like to try supplements, you should probably focus on those that have been shown help reduce fibromyalgia symptoms in some patients.

Doctors use medical research to help them decide if treatments are likely to be safe and effective for you. Research studies testing many treatments for fibromyalgia (like exercise, behavioral therapy, and medications) have used very rigorous testing methods to prove that these treatments are effective. These therapies have been tested in many studies testing large groups of patients. These studies have shown that these therapies work better than taking a sugar pill or placebo. While a number of studies have also tested nutritional supplements, these studies have usually used a small number of patients and the supplements usually have not tested treatments against a placebo. Also, in many cases, only one or two studies have been done with each individual supplement. For these reasons, doctors do not have as much information about whether supplements are likely to be helpful for you or not.

A number of research studies have tested which supplements are likely to help reduce fibromyalgia symptoms. Although the information is limited, using the information from these studies can help suggest supplements that are more likely to reduce fibromyalgia symptoms. Those treatments that have been shown to help fibromyalgia patients include:

- Vitamin C 500–1,000 mg daily
- Vitamin D replacement when blood levels of vitamin D levels are tested as low; vitamin D dose will depend on your level of vitamin D deficiency
- S-adenosyl methionine, also called SAMe, 800 mg daily
- Melatonin 3 mg taken 30 min before bed
- Fresh water alga Chlorella pyrenoidosa 10 mg tablet plus 100 mL liquid daily
- Coenzyme Q10 100–200 mg daily
- Carnitine 1,000–1,500 mg daily
- Fish oil 1,500 mg three times daily

Some studies suggest that the following treatments *may* be helpful, but studies testing them in fibromyalgia patients have not been done:

- Magnesium
- Probiotics for digestive symptoms
- Zinc

Always talk to your healthcare provider before taking any supplement and let him or her know what supplement you are currently using.

References

1. Bennett RM, Friend R, Jones KD, et al. The revised fibromyalgia impact questionnaire (FIQR): validation and psychometric properties. Arthritis Res Ther. 2009;11:R120.
2. Parker G, Hilton T, Bains J, Hadzi-Pavlovic D. Cognitive-based measures screening for depression in the medically ill: the DMI-10 and the DMI-18. Acta Psychiatr Scand. 2002;105:419–26.
3. Spitzer RL, Kroenke K, Williams JW, Löwe B. A brief measure for assessing generalized anxiety disorder. The GAD-7. Arch Intern Med. 2006;166:1092–7.
4. Wallston KA, Wallston BS, DeVellis R. Health Educ Monog. 1978;6:160–70.
5. Wallston KA, Stein MJ, Smith CA. J Pers Assess. 1994;63:534–53.

Part IV
Special Populations

Fibromyalgia and Pregnancy

Key Chapter Points

- Fibromyalgia symptoms tend to worsen with menstrual periods, pregnancy, and delivery.
- Pregnancy outcome is unaffected by a fibromyalgia diagnosis.
- Pre-conception discussions should be a routine part of the care of fibromyalgia patients of childbearing potential.
- Nausea should be treated aggressively during pregnancy to avoid dehydration and poor nutrition.
- Non-drug treatments should be maximized during pregnancy and when nursing, with medications reserved for more disabling and recalcitrant symptoms.

Keywords Breastfeeding · Delivery · Nursing · Pregnancy · Post-partum

Case: Tiffany is 26 years old with fibromyalgia. "When I first found out I was pregnant, I was SO happy. I'd planned to avoid all medications with my pregnancy. My best friend gets terrible migraines and she told me how she had no migraines during pregnancy. I thought my fibromyalgia might get better too, but it just got worse and worse throughout the pregnancy. My doctor wouldn't give me anything and I felt so guilty just praying I'd have the baby early."

Although fibromyalgia is more prevalent in women, including women of child-bearing age, little is written about fibromyalgia and pregnancy. Pregnancy is a symptom-producing condition and often affects chronic pain syndromes, like fibromyalgia. Concerns about possible harmful effects from medical treatments on the developing baby may result in healthcare providers opting to take a wait-and-see approach with pregnancy – hoping that fibromyalgia symptoms may improve or

D.A. Marcus, A. Deodhar, *Fibromyalgia*, DOI 10.1007/978-1-4419-1609-9_16,
© Springer Science+Business Media, LLC 2011

abate so that treatment is unnecessary during fetal development with pregnancy and post-partum when breastfeeding. Although few studies have explored pregnancy-related issues in fibromyalgia patients, those studies that are available offer practical advice for healthcare providers and their fibromyalgia patients.

> **Case:** Tiffany also struggled with nursing. "Once Tyler was born, I couldn't wait to start nursing. I know it's so good for the baby and a great way to help lose the extra weight I'd gained during my pregnancy. Breastfeeding was such a struggle. I could never get comfortable and every time I tried to change my position, the baby lost interest in nursing. He always seemed hungry and I think I was too stressed out to make enough milk. After a month, I just gave up, but I feel so sad about nursing such a short time when I'd planned to nurse for at least 6 months."

Epidemiology of Fibromyalgia During Pregnancy

The effect of hormonal changes on fibromyalgia symptoms in women was evaluated in a small but important study in Norway [1]. Associations between different hormonal stages and overall fibromyalgia status were evaluated in 26 women. In this study, fibromyalgia symptoms worsened for most women in connection with their menstrual periods, pregnancy, and delivery (Fig. 1).

> **Practical pointer**
>
> At least three of every four fibromyalgia patients reported symptom worsening with menstrual periods, pregnancy, and delivery.

Fibromyalgia and Pregnancy

In the important Norwegian study described above, the effect of pregnancy on fibromyalgia was evaluated by comparing 40 pregnancies occurring in women who had fibromyalgia at the time of their pregnancies with 41 pregnancies that occurred in women who experienced fibromyalgia symptoms only after they had already completed their childbearing [1]. In general, pregnancy outcome was similar for women with and without fibromyalgia at the time of their pregnancies, with both groups tending to have normal pregnancies and healthy babies. Fibromyalgia symptoms, however, were most likely to worsen during pregnancy, with symptoms most severe during the third trimester (Fig. 2). The most commonly reported

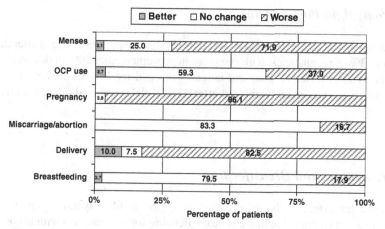

Fig. 1 Effect of hormonal events on fibromyalgia symptoms (based on Ostensen [1]). OCP=oral contraceptive

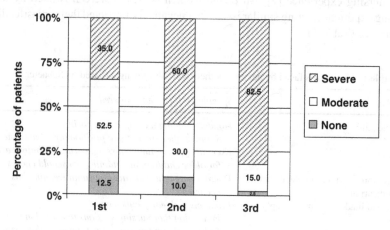

Fig. 2 Severity of fibromyalgia symptoms during each trimester of pregnancy (based on Ostensen [1])

fibromyalgia symptom during pregnancy was generalized pain (58% of patients), although women also reported fatigue, joint pain, back pain, depression, weakness, stiffness, and disability.

Practical pointer

Patients with fibromyalgia have no increased risk of miscarriage or complicated pregnancy.

Fibromyalgia Post-partum

In the Norwegian study reported above, fibromyalgia symptoms changed after delivery for 93% of pregnancies, with symptom improvement after 10% of deliveries and worsening after 83% [1]. Pain and fatigue worsened for 58% of mothers 1 month after delivery. Depression worsened after 43% of deliveries and anxiety increased for 18%.

Fibromyalgia and Breastfeeding

Although breastfeeding is not expected to aggravate fibromyalgia symptoms for most women [1], breastfeeding can be challenging for new mothers with fibromyalgia. A small, but important study surveyed nine women with fibromyalgia about their nursing experience [2]. All of the women surveyed were frustrated by their nursing experience, citing similar issues that negatively impacted their breastfeeding experience (Table 1).

Table 1 Challenges faced by nursing mothers with fibromyalgia (based on Schaefer [4])

Problem	Specific problems encountered
Muscle pain	Difficulty finding a comfortable position
	Stiffness after staying in a position for a long time
Fatigue	Excessive fatigue limits nursing, caring for baby, caring for older children, maintaining household chores
Restrictions from taking necessary medications	Doctors may refuse medications until weaning has occurred
Perceived inadequate milk supply	Problems with early milk supply
	Perception that nursing sessions took too long
	Concern that baby was not getting enough nutrition
Guilt and depression about unplanned early weaning	Perceptions of being an inadequate mother after abandoning nursing prior to initial intentions

Treating Fibromyalgia Throughout Pregnancy

Women with fibromyalgia may be less likely to choose to conceive. In an interesting study, fecundity was evaluated in patients with temporomandibular dysfunction (TMD) due to myofascial abnormalities [3]. Fecundity, or number of offspring, may be related to fertility issues as well as choice to start or add to families. In this study, those TMD patients with co-morbid fibromyalgia had fewer offspring than TMD patients without fibromyalgia or healthy controls (Fig. 3). There was no increase

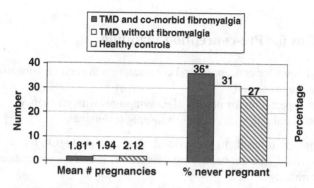

Fig. 3 Fecundity in patients with myofascial temporomandibular dysfunction (TMD) (based on Raphael [3]). Significant difference from controls: *$P < 0.05$

in menstrual irregularities or problems conceiving among fibromyalgia patients to explain the fewer pregnancies and offspring. While there were no differences in fertility factors, women with fibromyalgia did note that they were more likely to choose not to have children.

While some women with fibromyalgia will select not to start families, a number of your fibromyalgia patients will have pregnancy concerns. Directly addressing pregnancy-related concerns and offering practical advice for treating fibromyalgia symptoms throughout each stage of pregnancy can help reduce patient fears and facilitate a more successful pregnancy experience [4].

Pre-conception Planning

All women of childbearing potential should be regularly asked about current contraception and plans for conception. Women considering conceiving should be informed about the possibility of worsening symptoms, including pain and fatigue, during pregnancy, and a plan for treating fibromyalgia symptoms during pregnancy should be developed (Box 1). Because nausea is often particularly problematic during the early weeks of pregnancy, patients should also be provided with recommendations for treating nausea during pregnancy (Box 2).

The pre-conception period is an ideal time for maximizing the use of effective non-medication treatments, like exercise, strength training, and pain management skills. Patients previously trained in these techniques may benefit from booster sessions to help reinforce and hone skills. Patients should be encouraged to utilize these skills throughout the period of attempted conception and pregnancy. Medications that should be avoided during pregnancy should also be tapered and discontinued at this time, if possible.

Box 1 Tips for Pre-conception Planning

- Discuss plans for conception and contraception at each visit for women of childbearing potential
- Review expectation for fibromyalgia symptoms with pregnancy
- Maximize training with effective non-drug techniques

  - Consider referral to behavioral pain psychologist for cognitive-behavioral, operant-behavioral, relaxation, and stress management therapy training
  - Consider referral to physical therapy for development of effective aerobic and strength training exercise program
  - Consider referral to dietician for nutritional assistance in patients with gastrointestinal symptoms, such as irritable bowel syndrome
  - Reinforce sleep hygiene techniques

- Prescribe daily multivitamin with at least 400 micrograms of folate
- Review medications and develop a treatment plan that the patient can use when trying to conceive and when pregnant

Box 2 Tips for Reducing Nausea During Pregnancy

- Drink small amounts of cold, clear, carbonated drinks between meals. Try ginger ale or lemon-lime soda, clear broth, juice diluted with water, gelatin, electrolyte drinks (e.g., Gatorade and Pedialyte), and popsicles.
- Eat in a quiet, well ventilated, cool room.
- Slowly eat small portions of easily tolerated foods, like bananas, applesauce, rice, toast.
- Eat frequent small meals and healthy snacks as an empty stomach can aggravate nausea.
- Eggs and yogurt are good sources of protein and nutrition.
- Choose salty foods instead of sweets. Avoid spicy, fried, or fatty foods.
- Keep a tin of crackers at your bedside. Eat a few crackers before getting up in the morning.
- If odors increase your nausea, try frozen or prepared foods to reduce cooking.

Pregnancy

Fibromyalgia patients should be reminded to continue to utilize effective non-medication treatments, like low-impact aerobics, strength training exercises, pain management skills (like cognitive-behavioral, operant-behavioral, and relaxation therapies), and sleep hygiene techniques. Specific guidance about the safe use of non-drug treatments during pregnancy should be provided to patients to encourage utilization of effective, pain-relieving, non-medication therapies.

> **Practical pointer**
>
> Pain management during pregnancy should focus on utilization of effective, non-medication treatments due to the generally modest benefit and potential for side effects with many standard fibromyalgia medications.

Most doctors and patients would ideally like to avoid medications during pregnancy, however, this is not always feasible. In the Norwegian study reported above, 89% of fibromyalgia patients believed that they needed drug treatment for fibromyalgia during pregnancy, although only 44% received medications [1]. The most commonly used medications were analgesics (44%), antidepressants (15%), and sedatives (7%). Because medications offer only modest efficacy, drug treatments should be reserved for those women with more disabling and recalcitrant symptoms. Proactive conversations about which medications are safer to use during pregnancy and which should be avoided should be a routine part of caring for the pregnant fibromyalgia patient, even in patients not currently using medications, to avoid unsafe use.

> **Practical pointer**
>
> Patients should be directly counseled about safer medication use and restrictions that are advised during pregnancy and when nursing.

Modifying Non-medication Treatments During Pregnancy

Psychological pain management skills (including cognitive-behavioral, operant-behavioral, and relaxation therapies) can be used the same during pregnancy as in the non-pregnant patient. Although not specifically tested in fibromyalgia patients, psychological pain management techniques have been shown to effectively reduce chronic pain symptoms during pregnancy [5, 6].

Pregnant fibromyalgia patients should also be encouraged to continue to exercise. The American College of Obstetricians and Gynecologists (ACOG) guidelines for exercise during pregnancy generally recommend at least 30 min of moderate physical activity on most days of the week, with active pregnant women encouraged to continue exercise and sedentary women advised to begin an exercise program [7]. Exercise will likely need to be restricted in women with risk factors for preterm labor or hypertension. Patients can access an ACOG-produced exercise instruction guide online [8]. Tips for exercising during pregnancy can also be found in Box 3. Aerobic activities for fibromyalgia treatment should be limited to low-impact exercises (e.g., walking or swimming); high-impact exercise or activities likely to be associated with falls or trauma should be avoided. The ACOG specifically recommends avoiding skiing, contact sports, horseback riding, gymnastics, and scuba diving during pregnancy [8]. A recent review of prospectively collected data in the Danish National Birth Cohort showed no adverse effects from swimming in pool water during pregnancy [9]. Indeed, the risks for preterm delivery (hazard ratio = 0.08, 95% confidence interval 0.72–0.88) and congenital malformations

---

Box 3 Patient Recommendations for Exercise During Pregnancy (Adapted from ACOG Recommendations [8])

- Talk to your doctor about starting a new exercise program when you are pregnant
- Plan to exercise at least 30 min most days each week
- Limit aerobic exercise to low-impact activities, like walking, biking, or swimming
- Avoid contact sports and exercise associated with likely falls or trauma
- Stay hydrated and drink a glass of water before and after each exercise session
- Avoid doing exercises lying on your back after the first trimester
- Avoid getting overheated while exercising or working out in hot, humid environments
- Be sure to add extra calories to your diet when you are exercising

- Wear comfortable clothing, a supportive bra, and athletic footwear for exercising
- Stop exercising and contact your doctor if any of the following occurs:

  - You feel dizzy, faint, or short of breath
  - You get headaches, chest pain, calf pain or swelling, or muscle weakness
  - You experience a decrease in your baby's movements
  - You notice leaking of vaginal fluid or bleeding
  - You feel contractions

(odds ratio = 0.89, 95% confidence interval 0.08–0.98) were slightly decreased for mothers who swam during pregnancy compared with non-exercisers. Modest strength training may also continue during pregnancy. Light resistance and toning exercises performed during the second and third trimesters were shown to have no negative effects on labor and delivery, newborn body size, or overall newborn health in 160 sedentary, pregnant women who were randomly assigned to exercise three times weekly for 35–40 min per session or a non-exercise control [10, 11]. Adequate hydration should be encouraged during exercise. In general, pregnant women are recommended to drink 8–10 glasses of water daily [12], with additional fluid taken before and after exercise sessions.

Practical pointer

Healthy patients with fibromyalgia should be encouraged to continue low-impact aerobics and modest strength exercises during pregnancy.

Massage has shown modest benefits for fibromyalgia; however, this soothing therapy may be preferentially offered as part of a more comprehensive non-medication treatment program during pregnancy when medication options are limited. Studies suggest that massage should be performed about once or twice weekly for fibromyalgia patients [13].

Reinforcing sleep hygiene strategies may be particularly important during pregnancy as pregnancy itself tends to aggravates sleep disturbances. A prospective survey of 325 women compared sleep patterns before pregnancy and during each trimester [14]. The following patterns were recorded pre-pregnancy and during the first, second, and third trimesters, respectively: total sleep 8.0, 8.7, 8.4, and 8.3 h; restless sleep 10.0, 15.4, 20.3, and 30.3%; no nighttime awakenings 27.2, 7.8, 5.5, and 1.9%. Although benefits from acupuncture for reducing symptoms during pregnancy are generally inconclusive [15], a small, prospective, controlled study ($N=20$ enrolled with 12 completing the study) reported benefits from acupuncture in reducing insomnia during pregnancy.

Safety Rating Systems

The relative safety of drug therapy during pregnancy has been rated in several systems. The most widely used tool in the United States is the Food and Drug Administration (FDA) safety rating system, which rates medication risk based on the available data in human and animal studies. Clinicians generally agree that drugs in FDA risk categories A and B are relatively safe and those in categories D and X should be limited. The majority of medications, however, are classified as the more

Table 2 FDA pregnancy safety ratings (based on Uhl [16])

FDA risk	Safety	2001 PDR N = 2,249 drugs (%)	2002 PDR N = 2,150 drugs (%)
A	Established as safe	0.2	0.3
B	Likely to be safe	13	14
C	Teratogenicity possible	37	37
D	Teratogenicity probable	4	4
X	Teratogenicity likely	5	6
None listed	No information	41	39

nebulous category C, meaning adequate data are not available and teratogenicity is possible. Clinicians are generally advised to consider using category C drugs only when treatment benefits are considered to outweigh possible risks. Table 2 shows FDA pregnancy risk category assignment for drugs in the 2001 and 2002 Physicians' Desk References. Over 60% of those drugs assigned to a pregnancy risk class were categorized as C [16].

Safety during pregnancy is also assessed through the Teratogen Information System (TERIS), which catalogs risk of teratogenic effects for the offspring of exposed women as none, minimal, small, moderate, or high. When no or limited human data are available, a drug is classified as having an undetermined risk. An unlikely rating is given when risk is considered to probably be very low, however supportive data are limited. Using the TERIS system, 91% of drugs assessed in 2002 were considered to have undetermined pregnancy risk [17].

Clinical applicability of pregnancy risk rating systems is further limited by poor agreement among different safety rating systems. In an interesting study, pregnancy risk category assignment was compared for drugs common to three different classification systems: the United States FDA, the Australian Drug Evaluation Committee (ADEC), and the Swedish Catalogue of Approved Drugs (FASS) [18]. Only one in four of the drugs common to all three systems received the same risk factor category (Table 3). Differences were attributed to disparity in definitions among the three systems, as well as dissimilarities in the way accessible literature was used to determine risk category.

Table 3 Pregnancy risk category assignment for 236 drugs common to three international systems, N (%) (based on Addis [18] and reprinted with permission. Marcus and Bain. *Effective Migraine Treatment in Pregnant and Lactating Women.* Springer 2009)

Risk category	FDA	ADEC	FASS
A	6 (2.5)	50 (21.2)	59 (25.0)
B	62 (26.3)	71 (30.1)	65 (27.2)
C	115 (48.7)	84 (35.6)	85 (36.0)
D	45 (19.1)	29 (12.3)	27 (11.4)
X	8 (3.4)	2 (0.8)	Not used

Due to recognized problems with currently available rating systems, the FDA has proposed eliminating their current letter rating system in favor of providing more detailed text sections detailing pregnancy safety for each drug. Descriptive passages might include more extensive information about available data, information about whether data are from animal or human studies, and contrasting risks and benefits from drug exposure. In addition, the FDA recently formed a collaboration with 11 health plan-affiliated research sites to collect outcome data with prescription drug use during pregnancy in the Medication Exposure in Pregnancy Risk Evaluation Program (MEPREP), which will hopefully provide additional needed information on drug safety drug pregnancy.

Analgesics

Acetaminophen is considered to be relatively safe to use during pregnancy. Large epidemiological studies show no long-term effects in exposed babies [19].

Early NSAID exposure has been linked to increased risk for miscarriage. A post hoc analysis of retrospectively collected data reported an 80% increased risk of miscarriage among NSAID users, with risk highest when NSAIDs were used around the time of conception [20]. In this same report, paracetamol (acetaminophen) use was not linked to increased miscarriage risk. While NSAIDs are generally restricted only during the third trimester in the United States, their use is limited to the second trimester in many European countries. Recent recommendations from the European Federation of Neurological Societies advised use of acetaminophen/paracetamol throughout pregnancy, with NSAIDs restricted to the second trimester [21].

Aspirin is generally restricted during pregnancy, however, women who have inadvertently used aspirin in early pregnancy can be comforted by data from a meta-analysis of the literature and a large epidemiological study using national registry data in Hungary, both of which showed no increased risk of congenital malformations among the offspring of women using aspirin during the first trimester [22, 23]. Furthermore, a large epidemiological study of 19,226 pregnancies showed no negative long-term effects on intellectual development in 4-year olds who had been exposed to aspirin during their first 20 weeks of gestation [24].

Opioids should be used very infrequently for fibromyalgia in general, although they have a long track record of use for treating a variety of pain complaints during pregnancy and are generally considered to be safe during pregnancy [25–27]. Patients using opioids during pregnancy should be frequently and carefully monitored to minimize opioid overuse. Patients chronically using daily opioids during mid-to-late pregnancy should continue daily opioids for the duration of pregnancy because of the risks of fetal mortality and premature labor associated with intrauterine fetal opioid withdrawal [28]. The labor staff will need to be notified if opioids have been used in late pregnancy so the newborn can be assessed for sedation and possible opioid withdrawal.

Practical pointer

Acetaminophen may be used throughout pregnancy. NSAIDs are best limited to use in the second trimester.

Antidepressants

Most antidepressants are FDA risk category C drugs, while paroxetine is category D. In comparison to exposure with other antidepressants, paroxetine monotherapy in the first trimester has been linked to a modestly increased risk of congenital malformations (odds ratio = 1.89, 95% confidence interval 1.20–2.98) [29]. In one study, paroxetine exposure during the first trimester was linked to an increased risk of major malformations (odds ratio = 2.2) and major cardiac malformations (odds ratio = 3.1) only among women using a daily dosage >25 mg [30]. A prospective comparison of the offspring from 928 women exposed to antidepressants during the first trimester and 928 matched controls showed no difference in occurrence of major malformations with antidepressant exposure (3.2% vs. 3.3%) [31]. Miscarriage, however, was linked to antidepressant use in a meta-analysis that included women using antidepressants ($N = 1,534$) and non-depressed women ($N = 2,033$) [32]. Miscarriage occurred more frequently in the depressed women treated with antidepressants (12% vs. 4%, relative risk = 1.45). No differences were found among antidepressant drug classes. Furthermore, these data did not clarify whether the increased miscarriage rate was due to depression-related factors or medication use. A recent meta-analysis reported higher miscarriage risks with paroxetine [Paxil] (odds ratio 1.7, 95% confidence interval [CI] 1.3–2.3) and venlafaxine [Effexor] (odds ratio = 2.1, 95% CI 1.3–3.3) [33].

Serotonin reuptake inhibitors exposure during pregnancy has been linked to an increased risk for low birth weight, respiratory distress, persistent pulmonary hypertension in the newborn, and miscarriage [34, 35]. A recent report on duloxetine [Cymbalta] exposure during pregnancy reported outcome from 12 babies exposed to duloxetine in utero, with no identified problems except for one case of neonatal behavioral syndrome [36]. Serotonin reuptake inhibitors (selective serotonin reuptake inhibitors [SSRIs] and serotonin and norepinephrine reuptake inhibitors) readily cross the placenta and increase central serotonergic tone in the developing fetus, with third trimester exposure linked to neonatal behavioral syndrome [37, 38]. In comparison to babies with no in utero exposure to serotonin reuptake inhibitors or exposure during early pregnancy, babies exposed in the third trimester carry a risk ratio of 3.0 for developing neonatal behavioral syndrome. Features typically include tremors/jitteriness, increased muscle tone/reflexes, feeding/digestive disturbances, irritability/agitation, respiratory disturbances, excessive crying, and sleep disturbances. In most cases, symptoms are mild and respond to supportive measures. Possible long-term effects of changes in in utero serotonergic tone have not been studied [37].Third trimester treatment with either tricyclic or SSRI antidepressants has been linked to increased perinatal complications, including respiratory distress, endocrine and metabolic disorders, and temperature regulation disturbances [39]. Interestingly, discontinuing SSRI exposure during the third trimester does not appear to improve neonatal outcome [40].

Practical pointer

Antidepressants may be necessary to treat severe mood disorders during pregnancy. Antidepressants, however, are infrequently recommended for pain management during pregnancy, due to small risks identified with most groups of antidepressants in both early and late pregnancy.

Antiepileptics

Both pregabalin and gabapentin are FDA pregnancy risk category C drugs. Limited data are available on the safety of either drug during pregnancy, with some data reported in the literature for gabapentin [41]. Gabapentin is thought to be actively transported by the placenta with accumulation in the fetus [42]. Small studies in epileptic women have not identified fetal effects with gabapentin treatment [43]. A review of available data from the UK National Teratology Information Service identified no increased malformation risk with gabapentin [44]. The Gabapentin Pregnancy Registry published data on 44 live births, with no increased risk of miscarriage, low birth weight, or malformation seen in gabapentin-exposed babies [45]. The very small number in this sample, however, substantially limits safety interpretations that can be made using these data. Recently, data from the Swedish Medical Birth Registry showed no effect on head circumference in newborns who had been exposed to gabapentin ($N = 69$) [46]. When gabapentin is used during pregnancy for pain management, it is typically discontinued in the third trimester because of possible interference with bony development.

Information for patients exposed to antiepileptics during pregnancy in the United States is being collected through the North American Antiepileptic Drug (NAAED) Pregnancy Registry at http://www.aedpregnancyregistry.org/. Patients exposed can participate in this registry by contacting 1-888-233-2334. Data for exposures in Europe, Australia, and South American can be provided to the International Registry of Antiepileptic Drugs and Pregnancy (EURAP; http://www.eurapinternational. org).

Sodium Oxybate

Narcolepsy drug, sodium oxybate, which has demonstrated benefit in fibromyalgia (see chapter "Medication Treatments") is an FDA risk category B drug. As limited data are available on using this drug during pregnancy, it should probably be limited to patients with recalcitrant and severe symptoms in whom possible risks are outweighed by expected benefits.

Anti-emetics

Nausea can be particularly problematic during pregnancy for women with fibromyalgia. Encourage woman to follow the nausea prevention tips provided during pre-conception counseling (Box 2). Persistent nausea should be treated aggressively to avoid dehydration and poor nutrition (Fig. 4). The most commonly recommended treatments by practicing obstetricians for pregnancy-related nausea include nutritional supplements and behavioral therapy [47], which are most effective for mild nausea. Moderate-to-severe nausea and/or vomiting will likely need to be treated with medications, such as metoclopramide, ondansetron, or promethazine.

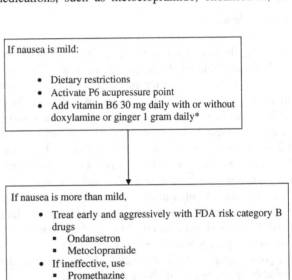

Fig. 4 Recommendations for treatment of nausea during conception and pregnancy (reprinted with permission. Marcus and Bain. *Effective Migraine Treatment in Pregnant and Lactating Women.* Springer 2009). *Most studies have evaluated safety when using either supplement for 3–4 days. One study treated patients daily for 3 weeks, with good safety

If nausea is mild:

- Dietary restrictions
- Activate P6 acupressure point
- Add vitamin B6 30 mg daily with or without doxylamine or ginger 1 gram daily*

If nausea is more than mild,

- Treat early and aggressively with FDA risk category B drugs
  - Ondansetron
  - Metoclopramide
- If ineffective, use
  - Promethazine
  - Combination therapy

Labor and Delivery

Labor should occur in a cool, quiet, calm environment with minimal unnecessary stimulation. Encourage fibromyalgia patients to walk and change positions frequently during labor, as possible. Ask the nursing staff to help patients practice relaxation techniques during labor and provide heat and counterpressure to the sacrum [4].

Post-delivery fibromyalgia treatment should include discussions of plans for contraception. Contraception after delivery can be achieved with condoms, spermicides, and/or an intrauterine device. Combined hormonal contraceptives are not recommended during the immediate post-partum period, while progestin-only preparations may be used. Furthermore, estrogen is associated with reduced milk production [48].

Safety Determinations with Breastfeeding

In 2001, the American Academy of Pediatrics published classifications of common drugs based on compatibility with breastfeeding [49]. Both the American Academy of Pediatrics (http://aappolicy.aappublications.org/) and the World Health Organization (WHO, http://www.who.int/child-adolescent-health/) provide online resources cataloguing drug safety. Additional information about drug use during lactation can be found online at the Drugs and Lactation Database (LactMed at http://toxnet.nlm.nih.gov/), managed by the United States National Library of Medicine. Information may also be obtained from a Web site managed by Thomas W. Hale, RPh, PhD, Professor of Pediatrics at Texas Tech University (http://neonatal.ttuhsc.edu/lact/).

Analgesics

Analgesics considered to be compatible with nursing include acetaminophen, ibuprofen, and naproxen [50, 51]. Ibuprofen has poor transfer to breast milk [52] and its use in children is well documented. Other nonsteroidal anti-inflammatory drugs (NSAIDs, e.g., naproxen [Naprosyn, Aleve], piroxicam [Feldene], and sulindac [Clinoril]), are excreted into the breast milk and have undesirable longer half-lives that may result in drug accumulation with repeat dosing. The American Academy of Pediatrics lists naproxen as compatible with breastfeeding, although data supporting this classification are less abundant than with ibuprofen [49].

Infrequently administered opioids can be used; however, repeated dosing should be avoided and babies should be observed for apnea, bradycardia, and cyanosis. This caution is supported by a case report of an infant dying from morphine toxicity caused by repeated use of acetaminophen plus codeine by the nursing mother who was a cytochrome P450 CYP2D6 ultra-rapid metabolizer [53]. Codeine is metabolized to morphine via CYP2D6 and newborns have a reduced capacity to metabolize and eliminate morphine. Duplications of CYP2D6 genes can result in ultra-rapid drug metabolism. These duplications occur in 1% of Caucasian Americans, 65.8% of African-Americans, and 2% of racially mixed Americans [54]. The occurrence of rapid metabolizers among a minority of breastfeeding mothers would result in an increased requirement for codeine in these patients to achieve analgesic effect and subsequent exposure to unexpectedly high morphine concentrations in their breastfed infants.

Practical pointer

Single doses of opioids are safe when nursing. Repeated doses, especially when taken by women who are rapid metabolizers, can be problematic and should be avoided.

Fibromyalgia patients with migraine may use sumatriptan when nursing [49]. Sumatriptan is minimally excreted into breast milk, with only 0.24% of the maternal dosage recovered in breast milk [55].

Antidepressants

Antidepressants are excreted into breast milk and their effects on the baby's developing nervous system are unknown. Duloxetine concentration in the breast milk is about $\frac{1}{4}$ the concentration seen in maternal plasma [56]. The Academy of Breastfeeding Medicine Protocol Committee recently published guidelines governing the use of antidepressants in nursing mothers [57], with antidepressants recommended only for women with moderate–severe depressive symptoms. Sertraline was recommended as first-line antidepressant therapy, due to lower levels in breast milk and infant serum.

Practical pointer

Antidepressants are typically restricted when nursing to the treatment of moderate to severe depression due to unknown long-term effects on the developing baby's nervous system.

Sodium Oxybate

Data on excretion of sodium oxybate into breast milk are not available. Therefore, this drug should generally be restricted when nursing.

Antiepileptics

Information on the effects of neuromodulating antiepileptics on nursing babies is limited. The transfer of gabapentin to breast milk is substantial; however, plasma concentrations in nursing infants are low, with no adverse effects reported in exposed infants in the literature [42, 58]. Because of the limited literature available on pregabalin and gabapentin during pregnancy, use of these drugs should generally be limited when nursing.

Planning for Nursing Success

The American Academy of Pediatrics recommends breastfeeding exclusively during the baby's first 6 months of life, with additional nursing recommended for at least the baby's first year of life. Breastfeeding imparts important nutrition, hormones, and growth and immune factors to the baby, as well as facilitating return to normal maternal weight, reducing maternal risk for breast and ovarian cancers, and reducing risk for maternal rheumatoid arthritis [59, 60].

Plans for nursing should be initially addressed during the beginning of the third trimester of pregnancy (Box 4). Openly discussing common problems and suggestions for proactively addressing problems may improve satisfaction with the nursing process and improve success with breastfeeding.

Box 4 Tips for Successful Nursing

- At the beginning of the third trimester

  - Set up realistic expectations for nursing and fibromyalgia treatment options
  - Discuss expectations for fibromyalgia symptoms post-partum
  - Provide booster sessions with pain psychologist for pain management skills
  - Refer patient to lactation counselor
  - Assess mood and address, as appropriate

- Prior to delivery

  - Talk about prioritizing and scheduling essential chores for baby and the family after delivery
  - Include patient's support network in post-partum discussions
  - Help patient delegate chores to support network members
  - Reinforce nutritional goals
  - Review expectations for increased fatigue post-partum
  - Assess mood and address, as appropriate
  - Review treatment plans for after delivery

- Prior to hospital discharge after delivery

  - Congratulate patient on her decision to nurse and remind her that the baby gets important health benefits even if she is not able to nurse for as long as she would like.
  - Remind patient to find comfortable positions when nursing, such as nursing lying on her side or using a pillow or sling to help support the weight of the baby
  - Remind patient to change positions frequently during nursing sessions to reduce getting sore and stiff
  - Encourage patient to nurse baby in a quiet, comfortable environment
  - Contact patient's lactation counselor and arrange for follow-up contact
  - Review treatment plan for fibromyalgia symptoms
  - Schedule follow-up to assess patient's fibromyalgia symptoms soon after discharge

Summary

- Fibromyalgia symptoms tend to worse during pregnancy, with over 80% of women reporting severe fibromyalgia symptoms during the third trimester.
- Although nursing per se does not aggravate overall fibromyalgia symptoms, nursing can provide unique challenges for the fibromyalgia patient that may limit success with continued nursing.
- Fibromyalgia patients should focus on maximizing effective non-drug treatments before conceiving, with plans to continue these treatments during pregnancy and with nursing.
- Patients should be reminded about the modest benefits expected from most medication treatments of fibromyalgia, with medications reserved for more disabling and recalcitrant symptoms that have failed to respond to non-drug therapies.
- Miscarriage risk increases with early exposures to nonsteroidal anti-inflammatory drugs and at least some antidepressants.
- Antidepressants are best reserved during pregnancy and nursing for patients with significant mood disorders that require medications.
- Safety data with neuromodulating antiepileptics are limited. Small samples have not identified problems with gabapentin in early pregnancy or when nursing.
- Sodium oxybate is an FDA pregnancy risk category B drug.

References

1. Ostensen M, Rugelsjøen A. Wigers Sh. The effect of reproductive events and alterations of sex hormone levels on the symptoms of fibromyalgia. Scand J Rheumatol. 1997;26:355–60.
2. Schaefer KM. Breastfeeding in chronic illness: the voices of women with fibromyalgia. MCN Am J Matern Child Nurs. 2004;29:248–53.

3. Raphael KG, Marbach JJ. Comorbid fibromyalgia accounts for reduced fecundity in women with myofascial face pain. Clin J Pain. 2000;16:29–36.

4. Schaefer KM, Black K. Fibromyalgia and pregnancy. What nurses need to know and do. AWHONN Lifelines. 2005;9:228–35.

5. Marcus DA, Scharff L, Turk DC. Nonpharmacological management of headaches during pregnancy. Psychosom Med. 1995;57:527–35.

6. Scharff L, Marcus DA, Turk DC. Maintenance of effects in the nonmedical treatment of headaches during pregnancy. Headache. 1996;36:285–90.

7. American College of Obstetricians and Gynecologists. Exercise during pregnancy and the postpartum period: Technical Bulletin 267. Washington, DC: ACOG Press, 2002.

8. http://www.acog.org/publications/patient_education/bp119.cfm. Accessed March 2010.

9. Juhl M, Kogevinas M, Andersen PK, Andersen AM, Olsen J. Is swimming during pregnancy a safe exercise? Epidemiology. 2010;21:253–8.

10. Barakat R, Ruiz JR, Stirling JR, Zakynthinaki M, Lucia A. Type of delivery is not affected by light resistance and toning exercise training during pregnancy: a randomized controlled trial. Am J Obstet Gynecol. 2009;201:590.

11. Barakat R, Lucia A, Ruiz JR. Resistance exercise training during pregnancy and newborn's birth size: a randomised controlled trial. Int J Obes. 2009;33:1048–57.

12. Montgomery KS. Nutrition column an update on water needs during pregnancy and beyond. J Perinat Educ. 2002;11:40–2.

13. Kalichman L. Massage therapy for fibromyalgia symptoms. Rheumatol Int. 2010;30:1151–7.

14. Hedman C, Pohjasvaara T, Tolonen U, Suhonen-Malm AS, Myllylä VV: Effects of pregnancy on mothers' sleep. Sleep Med. 2002;3:37–42.

15. Smith CA, Cochrane S. Does acupuncture have a place as an adjunct treatment during pregnancy? A review of randomized controlled trials and systematic reviews. Birth. 2009;36:246–53.

16. Uhl K, Kennedy DL, Kweder SL. Risk management strategies in the Physicians' Desk Reference product labels for pregnancy category X drugs. Drug Saf. 2002;25:885–92.

17. Lo WY, Firedman JM. Teratogenicity of recently introduced medications in human pregnancy. Obstet Gynecol. 2002;100:465–73.

18. Addis A, Sharabi S, Bonati M. Risk classification systems for drug use during pregnancy. Are they a reliable source of information? Drug Saf. 2000;23:245–53.

19. Streissguth AP, Treder RP, Barr HM, et al. Aspirin and acetaminophen use by pregnant women and subsequent child IQ and attention decrements. Teratology. 1987;35:211–9.

20. Li DK, Liu L, Odouli R. Exposure to non-steroidal anti-inflammatory drugs during pregnancy and risk of miscarriage: population based cohort study. BMJ. 2003;327:368.

21. Evers S, Áfra J, Frese A, et al. EFNS guideline on the drug treatment of migraine – report of an EFNS task force. Eur J Neurol. 2006;13:560–72.

22. Kozer E, Nikfar S, Costei A, et al. Aspirin consumption during the first trimester of pregnancy and congenital anomalies: a meta-analysis. Am J Obstet Gynecol. 2002;187:1623–30.

23. Nørgard B, Puhé E, Caeizel AE, Skriver MV, Sørensen HT. Aspirin use during early pregnancy and the risk of congenital abnormalities: a population-based case-control study. Am J Obstet Gynecol. 2005;192:922–3.

24. Klebanoff MA, Berendes HW. Aspirin exposure during the first 20 weeks of gestation and IQ at four years of age. Teratology. 1988;37:249–55.

25. Bracken MB, Holfod TR. Exposure to prescribed drugs in pregnancy and association with congenital malformations. Obstet Gynecol. 1981;58:336–44.

26. Saxén I. Epidemiology of cleft lip and palate. An attempt to rule out chance correlations. Br J Prev Soc Med. 1875;29:103–10.

27. Saxén I. Associations between oral clefts and drugs taken during pregnancy. Int J Epidemilol. 1975;4:37–44.

28. Beers MH, Berkow R, eds. Drug use and dependence. The Merck Manual of Diagnostics and Therapeutics, 17th ed., Section 15, Chapter 195. (Available at www.merck.com/pubs. Accessed September 30, 2007).

29. Cole JA, Ephross SA, Cosmatos JS, Walker AM. Paroxetine in the first trimester and the prevalence of congenital malformations. Pharmacoepidemiol Drug Saf. 2007;16: 1075–85.

30. Bérard A, Ramos E, Rey E, et al. First trimester exposure to paroxetine and risk of cardiac malformations in infants: the importance of dosage. Birth Defects Res B Dev Reprod Toxicol. 2007;80:18–27.

31. Einarson A, Choi J, Einarson TR, Koren G. Incidence of major malformations in infants following antidepressant exposure in pregnancy: results of a large prospective cohort study. Can J Psychiatry. 2009;54:242–6.

32. Hemels ME, Einarson A, Koren G, Lanctot KL, Einarson TR. Antidepressant use during pregnancy and the rates of spontaneous abortions: a meta-analysis. Ann Pharmacother. 2005;39:803–9.

33. Broy P, Bérard A. Gestational exposure to antidepressants and the risk of spontaneous abortion: a review. Curr Drug Deliv. 2010;7:76–92.

34. Oberlander TF, Warburton W, Misri A, Aghajanian J, Hertzman C. Neonatal outcomes after prenatal exposure to selective serotonin reuptake inhibitor antidepressants and maternal depression using population-based linked health data. Arch Gen Psychiatry. 2006;63: 898–906.

35. Tuccori M, Testi A, Antonioli L, et al. Safety concerns associated with the use of serotonin reuptake inhibitors and other serotonergic/noradrenergic antidepressants during pregnancy: a review. Clin Ther. 2009;31:1426–53.

36. Briggs GG, Ambrose PJ, Ilett KF, et al. Use of duloxetine in pregnancy and lactation. Ann Pharmacother. 2009;43:1898–902.

37. Oberlander TF, Gingrich JA, Ansorge MS. Sustained neurobehavioral effects of exposure to SSRI antidepressants during development: molecular to clinical evidence. Clin Pharmacol Ther. 2009;86:672–7.

38. Moses-Kolko EL, Bogen D, Perel J, et al. Neonatal signs after late in utero exposure to serotonin reuptake inhibitors: literature review and implications for clinical applications. JAMA. 2005;293:2372–83.

39. Davis RL, Rubanowice D, McPhillips H, et al. Risks of congenital malformations and perinatal events among infants exposed to antidepressant medications during pregnancy. Pharmacoepidemiol Drug Saf. 2007;16:1086–94.

40. Warburton W, Hertzman C, Oberlander TF. A register study of the impact of stopping third trimester selective serotonin reuptake inhibitor exposure on neonatal health. Acta Psychiatr Scand. 2010;121:471–9.

41. Pennell PB. Antiepileptic drugs during pregnancy: what is known and which AEDs seem to be safest? Epilepsia. 2008;49:43–55.

42. Ohman I, Vitols S, Tomson T. Pharmacokinetics of gabapentin during delivery, in the neonatal period, and lactation: does a fetal accumulation occur during pregnancy? Epilepsia. 2005;46:1621–4.

43. Montouris G. Gabapentin exposure in human pregnancy: results from the Gabapentin Pregnancy Registry. Epilepsy Behav. 2003;4:310–7.

44. UK National Teratology Information Service September 2007 report. http://toxbase.org/upload/Pregnancy%20pdfs/Gabapentin2007.pdf. Accessed January 2010.

45. Montouris G. Gabapentin exposure in human pregnancy: results from the Gabapentin Pregnancy Registry. Epilepsy Behav. 2003;4:310–7.

46. Almgren M, Källén B, Lavebratt C. Population-based study of antiepileptic drug exposure in utero – influence on head circumference in newborns. Seizure. 2009;18:672–5.

47. Power ML, Milligan LA, Schulkin J. Managing nausea and vomiting of pregnancy: a survey of obstetrician-gynecologists. J Reprod Med. 2007;52:922–8.

48. Kennedy KI. Post-partum contraception. Bailleres Clin Obste Gynaecol. 1996;10:25–41.

49. American Academy of Pediatric Committee on Drugs. The transfer of drugs and other chemicals into human milk. Pediatrics. 2001;108:776–89.

50. Risser A, Donovan D, Heintzman J, Page T. NSAID prescribing precautions. Am Fam Physician. 2009;80:1371–8.

51. Madadi P, Ross CJ, Hayden MR, et al. Pharmacogenetics of neonatal opioid toxicity following maternal use of codeine during breastfeeding: a case-control study. Clin Pharmacol Ther. 2009;85:31–5.

52. Davies NM. Clinical pharmacokinetics of ibuprofen. The first 30 years. Clin Pharmacokinet. 1998;34:101–54.

53. Koren G, Cairns J, Chitayat D, Gaedigk A, Leeder SJ. Pharmacogenetics of morphine poisoning in a breastfed neonate of a codeine-prescribed mother. Lancet. 2006;368:704.

54. Gaedigk A, Ndjontché L, Divakaran K, et al. Cytochrome P4502D6 (CYP2D6) gene locus heterogeneity: characterization of gene duplication events. Clin Pharmacol Ther. 2007;81:242–51.

55. Wojnar-Horton RE, Hackett LP, Yapp P, et al. Distribution and excretion of sumatriptan in human milk. Br J Clin Pharmacol. 1996;41:217–21.

56. Lobo ED, Loghin C, Knadler MP. Pharmacokinetics of duloxetine in breast milk and plasma of healthy postpartum women. Clin Pharmacokinet. 2008;47:103–9.

57. Academy of Breastfeeding Medicine Protocol Committee. ABM clinical protocol #18: use of antidepressants in nursing mothers. Breastfeed Med. 2008;3:44–52.

58. Kristensen JH, Ilett KF, Hackett LP, Kohan R. Gabapentin and breastfeeding: a case reports. J Hum Lact. 2006;22:426–8.

59. Ip S, Chung M, Raman G, et al. Breastfeeding and maternal and infant health outcomes in developed countries. Evid Rep Technol Assess (Full Rep). 2007;135:1–186.

60. Pikwer M, Bergström U, Nilsson JA, et al. Breast-feeding, but not oral contraceptives, is associated with a reduced risk of rheumatoid arthritis. Ann Rheum Dis. 2009;68:526–30.

Fibromyalgia in Seniors

Key Chapter Points

- The clinical features of fibromyalgia and impact from fibromyalgia are generally similar in older and younger patients.
- Elderly patients with fibromyalgia are often misdiagnosed with other rheumatologic conditions, including inflammatory and degenerative arthritis.
- Geriatric-specific pain assessment tools are often helpful for clarifying pain severity and impact in older patients.
- Fibromyalgia in seniors is best treated with a combination of exercise, cognitive pain management techniques, and medications, although drug selection and dosages used may need to be modified due to co-morbid illness and increased propensity to experience troublesome side effects.

Keywords Elderly · Geriatric · Pain faces · Pain thermometer · Senior

> **Case:** Doris is a 67-year-old retired nurse. "I finally retired and was looking forward to golfing and traveling with my husband, but I'm so tired and I ache all over. I've seen my doctor several times, but he keeps saying my joints are fine, so I don't have arthritis and I should just ignore anything that's not 'pain.' It's really more of an ache than a pain, so I'm trying to forget about it, but it's really holding me back and spoiling my retirement. My friends tell me that I'm just bored after retiring and using doctor visits to fill a void. After working as a nurse for 30 years, I have a lot better things to do than hang out in doctors' waiting rooms! When I read about fibromyalgia on the Internet, it sounded just like me, but my doctor says fibromyalgia's a young woman's disease and I'm too old to start having fibromyalgia now."

D.A. Marcus, A. Deodhar, *Fibromyalgia*, DOI 10.1007/978-1-4419-1609-9_17,
© Springer Science+Business Media, LLC 2011

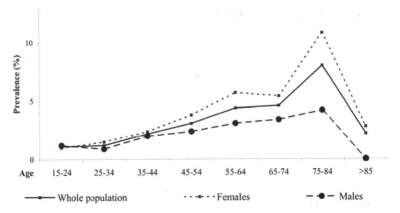

Fig. 1 Prevalence of fibromyalgia across age groups in a community sample (Reprinted with permission from Branco [3])

Fibromyalgia is most common among seniors, with more than 7% of women ≥ 60 years old affected [1]. In a Canadian survey, fibromyalgia prevalence peaked between ages 55 and 64 years old [2]. A recent population survey conducted in five European countries, likewise reported a relatively low prevalence in young adults, with prevalence increasing from ages 35 to 44 years through the senior years, with a sharp decline after age 84 years (Fig. 1) [3]. Subsequently, the prevalence of FM declined dramatically. Fibromyalgia, however, is often considered a condition of young adults, with seniors frequently misdiagnosed. In one study, only 17% of elderly patients with fibromyalgia had their condition recognized by their referring physicians [4]. In a comparable group of younger patients with fibromyalgia (<59 years old), fibromyalgia had been diagnosed in 26% of patients. Commonly assigned misdiagnoses in fibromyalgia patients ≥60 years old in this study were rheumatoid arthritis (27%), osteoarthritis (20%), "psychological" pain (10%), and polymyalgia rheumatica (6%). In addition, 40% of seniors with fibromyalgia had been treated with unnecessary corticosteroids prior to their eventual rheumatology referral.

Fibromyalgia symptoms, tender point examination, and disability are similar in seniors with fibromyalgia compared with younger fibromyalgia patients, although elderly patients tend to report milder symptom severity [4]. It is unclear if the difference in symptom severity reporting reflects milder symptoms in older patients or reduced self-reporting among seniors. Furthermore, fibromyalgia beginning after age 60 appears to be similar to fibromyalgia that begins in younger patients. A survey of 31 fibromyalgia patients ≥60 years old followed for up to 1 year after initial consultation showed similar outcome to that reported for younger patients [4]. Symptoms remained unchanged in 44%, somewhat worse in 11%, somewhat better in 15%, and moderately to much better in 30% after follow-up for a median of 6 months after initial rheumatologic consultation.

Fibromyalgia Assessment

Physical examination findings, including the presence of fibromyalgia tender points, have been shown to be both reliable and reproducible in seniors [5]. Similar to younger adults with fibromyalgia, seniors with fibromyalgia are expected to have a relatively unremarkable physical examination. It is important to ensure that widespread pain and somatic complaints are not caused by other medical conditions. Patients with abnormal examinations, especially the presence of true muscle weakness, will need to be thoroughly investigated for alternative diagnoses before a fibromyalgia diagnosis is given (Table 1).

Table 1 Assessing widespread pain and somatic complaints in seniors

Differential diagnosis	Recommended testing, especially in patients with true muscle weakness[a]
Ankylosing spondylitits or other arthritides	Complete blood count
Fibromyalgia	C-reactive protein or erythrocyte
Hypothyroidism	sedimentation rate
Hypovitaminosis D	Muscle enzymes, like creatinine kinase
Metastatic cancer	Serum protein electrophoresis
Multiple myeloma	Thyroid stimulating hormone
Polymyositis	Vitamin D 25(OH) level
Polymyalgia rheumatica	

[a]Additional testing should be guided based on patient history and physical examination findings

Specific recommendations for evaluating pain complaints in geriatric patients have been developed by the American Society of Geriatrics (Table 2) [6]. As illustrated by the case, descriptors used by seniors to describe pain may include seemingly benign terms, like "discomfort" and "ache" [7]. Pain in elderly patients should not be discounted because these apparently milder descriptors are selected.

> ## Practical pointer
>
> Do not discount reports of pain in older patients if they use descriptors like "ache," "discomfort," and "soreness" rather than pain.

Although the same general pain assessments used in younger patients may be applied to elderly patients, additional tools have been developed to allow convenient and appropriate assessment of pain severity and its impact in elderly populations. Replacing standard numeric rating or visual analogue pain scales with a pain thermometer or Faces Pain Scales may more effectively evaluate pain severity in older seniors (Fig. 2) [8]. Furthermore, assessment tools should be selected that

Table 2 Recommendations for assessing pain in seniors (based on AGS Panel [6])

Assessment	Specific recommendation
Identifying who to evaluate for pain	All seniors should be queried about possible pain complaints
Determining need for pain treatment	Pain impairing function of quality of life should be treated
Understanding pain severity	Seniors may select pain terms like "discomfort," "soreness," "heaviness," and "tightness" to describe significant pain
Evaluating patients with cognitive or language impairments	Evaluate vocalizations and nonverbal behavior. Query caregiver about functional impairments
Understanding pain complaint	Patients require a comprehensive history and physical examination, including assessment of co-morbid medical and psychological conditions and evaluation of functional disability
Consulting for additional services	Consider including pain management specialist for disabling, intractable pain, psychiatrist for depression, anxiety, or other severe psychiatric problems, and pain/addiction specialist for medication abuse/addiction concerns
Re-assessing patients	Regular reassessments are needed to evaluate symptom progression and treatment response

focus on disability for activities appropriate to the lifestyles of seniors. For example, questionnaires that query patients about work ability and caring for others in the household may not be relevant for many patients. Two geriatric assessment tools that incorporate both pain severity and associated disability are the Geriatric Pain Measure Questionnaire [9] (Table 3) and the 6-min walk test [10] (Box 1). The 6-min walk test is a practical measure of function that has been standardized in elderly patients. Results of both of these tests can be recorded in patient charting documentation to serve as anchor pre-treatment measures, with subsequent assessments used to evaluate and record treatment efficacy.

Practical pointer

The 6-min walk test is a practical and reproducible tool for monitoring important function in seniors.

Elderly patients with cognitive impairment provide unique challenges for pain management. Patient body language and vocalizations, as well as caregiver reports, can be used to help evaluate comfort level in these patients. Functional measures, including success with eating, sleeping, and activities of daily living, may also reflect pain impact.

(a)

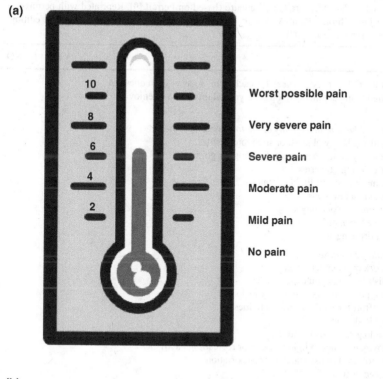

Worst possible pain

Very severe pain

Severe pain

Moderate pain

Mild pain

No pain

(b)

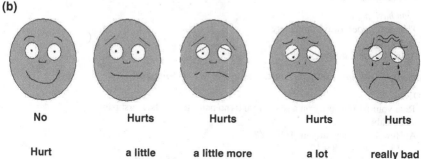

| No | Hurts | Hurts | Hurts | Hurts |
| Hurt | a little | a little more | a lot | really bad |

Fig. 2 Pain measures. (**a**) Pain thermometer, (**b**) pain faces

Fibromyalgia Treatment in Seniors

In general, the same non-medication and medication therapies used in younger adults are also used for seniors with fibromyalgia. As in younger fibromyalgia patients, seniors are also most likely to achieve a more satisfactory treatment response when non-medication therapies are used in addition to medications. Medication selection and dosing are more complicated in older patients because of the increased prevalence of co-morbid medical illness and increased sensitivity in seniors to medication side effects.

Table 3 Geriatric Pain Measure Questionnaire (based on Ferrell [9]. Reprinted with permission from Marcus DA. Chronic Pain. A Primary Care Guide to Practical Management, 2nd edition. Humana Press, Totowa, NJ, 2008)

	YES	NO

I. Please put a "YES" or "NO" check for each item. Answer each question considering the impact that PAIN has on your ability to do or enjoy activities

Do or would you have pain with any of the following activities
Running, lifting heavy objects, or strenuous sports
Moving a heavy table, vacuuming, bowling, or golfing
Lifting or carrying groceries
Climbing more than one flight of stairs
Climbing only a few steps
Walking more than one block
Walking one block or less
Bathing or dressing

Does or would pain cause you to
Reduce work or other activities
Accomplish less than you expect
Limit the type of work or activities you do
Use extra effort for work or other activities
Have trouble sleeping
Miss attending religious functions
Lack enjoyment in non-religious social or recreational activities
Be unable to travel or use standard transportation
Feel fatigued or tired

Do you have pain
That never goes away completely
Every day
At least several times a week

In the last week, has your pain caused you to feel sad or depressed
TOTAL
II. Rate your pain severity on a scale from 0 (no pain) to 10 (the worst pain imaginable)
  A. How severe is your pain TODAY?
     0 1 2 3 4 5 6 7 8 9 10
  B. What was your AVERAGE pain severity over the LAST WEEK?
     0 1 2 3 4 5 6 7 8 9 10

Scoring: Add total number of "YES" checks and two numbers from section II. Multiply sum by
            2.38 to produce a score ranging from 0 to 100
Interpretation: <30 is mild pain; 30–69 is moderate pain; >70 is severe pain

Non-medication Therapy

In general, elderly patients with chronic pain complaints respond well to non-drug therapies, including exercise (e.g., home-based exercise and Tai Chi) [11, 12] and psychological pain management skill training (e.g., cognitive-behavioral therapy,

Box 1 Six-minute Walking Test to Measure Function (Based on Enright [10])

- Mark a hallways with lines for every 100 feet or every half meter
- Ask your patient to walk back and forth in the hallway at a comfortable pace
- Allow rest breaks, as needed

- Calculate the total distance walked (including full and partial laps completed) over a 6-min period
- Mean distances walked for the average senior are as follows:

  - Men: 362 m or 1,188 feet
  - Women: 332 m or 1,089 feet

- Chart your patient's initial walking distance and then monitor for changes at subsequent visits

relaxation, and biofeedback) [13, 14]. For example, a 21-week strength training program in women with fibromyalgia (ages 60 ± 2 years old) resulted in about a 40% decrease in average pain severity [15]. Exercise recommendations may need to be adjusted due to co-morbid illness and baseline physical capabilities. Therapies that combine exercise and mind–body interventions, like T'ai Chi and Qi Gong, have demonstrated efficacy for reducing fibromyalgia symptoms and may be particularly attractive options for older seniors [16].

Exercise has additional beneficial effects for seniors overall for improving function. A longitudinal study evaluated the effect of regular exercise at least 4 days/week in patients ≥70 years old [17]. Elders participating in regular exercise at age 70 years were significantly more likely to be able to perform activities of daily living with ease at age 77 years than those who did not do regular exercise. This difference was still seen after adjusting for diabetes, hypertension, chronic back pain, loneliness, ease of performing ADLs at age 70 years, and health deterioration from age 70 to 77 years. Exercise is, therefore, an important recommendation for elderly patients to reduce pain and maximize long-term independence.

Practical pointer

Exercise is an important fibromyalgia treatment in seniors to reduce fibromyalgia symptoms and maintain functional ability.

Medications

While same medications used in younger adults are often used for fibromyalgia in elderly individuals, drug selection and dosage must be adjusted to minimize adverse events and drug interactions. A review of outpatient visits from two large national, ambulatory care surveys in the United States revealed the use of at least one inappropriate drug in elderly patients at 3.8% of visits [18]. The major categories of drug offenders were pain relievers and central nervous system drugs.

Antidepressants

Antidepressant may need to be used cautiously in seniors. A recent study identified an increase in white matter lesions on brain magnetic resonance scanning in elderly patients treated with antidepressants [19]. While the significance of this finding is unclear, these findings support limiting antidepressant exposure in non-depressed elder patients. In addition, elderly patients may be more susceptible to clinically significant hyponatremia when taking serotonin reuptake inhibitors [20].

Duloxetine has been shown to be both safe and effective for the treatment of depression and neuropathic pain in elderly patients [21, 22]. Treatment discontinuation due to side effects was more common in elderly patients treated with routine care, placebo, or duloxetine (Fig. 3). Elderly subpopulations with fibromyalgia show a similar clinical response with duloxetine to that seen in younger patients [23]. Milnacipran has also been used effectively for depression in patients with Alzheimer's disease [24]. Among patients with depression and Alzheimer's disease treated with milnacipran, somnolence was reported in 14% and mild hypomanic state in 14%, with symptoms resolving rapidly in all cases following dosage reduction or discontinuation. Tricyclic antidepressants (TCAs) are generally limited in elderly patients due to potential harmful side effects and poor tolerability. Trazodone [Desyrel] has fewer cardiovascular effects than TCAs and may be a better choice in seniors. Selective serotonin reuptake inhibitors (SSRIs) may be better tolerated that TCAs and SSRIs have not been linked to increased suicide risk in elderly patients [25].

Practical pointer

Duloxetine and milnacipran have been safely and effectively used in older patient samples.

Antiepileptics

Pregabalin and gabapentin have both been successfully used to treat postherpetic neuralgia in seniors [26]. A total of 106 patients $\geq$65 years old were included

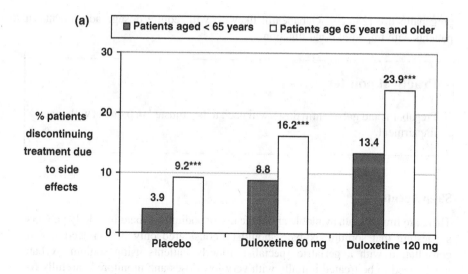

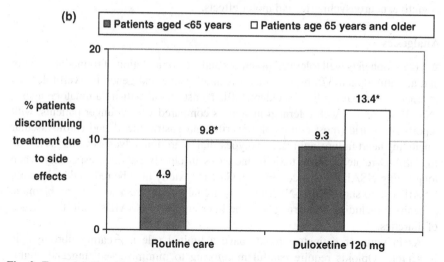

Fig. 3 Treatment discontinuation due to adverse events in duloxetine clinical trials (based on Wasan [22]). (**a**) Acute fibromyalgia treatment (12 weeks), (**b**) long-term extension (1 year). Significantly more patients ≥65 years old discontinued treatment due to adverse events with any treatment: $*P < 0.05$; $***P < 0.001$

in clinical trials with pregabalin and fibromyalgia [27]. Side effects were generally similar in older patients, although seniors were more likely to experience neurological side effects. Because pregabalin is excreted by the kidneys, dosage adjustments will be needed for elderly patients with co-morbid renal impairment. Furthermore, pregabalin should be used cautiously in patients with co-morbid heart failure patients as decompensation of chronic heart failure has been linked to pregabalin use [28, 29]. Gabapentin likewise will require dosage adjustments in patients with impaired renal function.

Practical pointer

Pregabalin and gabapentin doses will need to be adjusted in patients with renal impairment.

Sleep Agents

There are limited data available about the use of sodium oxybate in elderly patients, suggesting that sodium oxybate should be considered only in conjunction with consultation with a geriatric specialist. Elderly patients using sodium oxybate would need to be treated initially with very low doses and monitored carefully for cognitive, neuropsychiatric, and motor effects.

Analgesics

Acetaminophen is well tolerated in seniors and the combination of tramadol 37.5 mg and acetaminophen 325 mg [Ultracet] is an effective and generally well-tolerated alternative for pain relief in elders [30]. Nonsteroidal anti-inflammatory agents (NSAIDs) are less well tolerated in seniors compared with younger patients, with reports of gastric (most commonly gastritis and gastric ulcer) and cardiovascular (including heart failure, angina, and myocardial infarction) adverse events [31]. Risk for NSAID-related gastric toxicity increases in elderly patients, especially when long-acting NSAIDs are used [32, 33]. Gastric toxicity may be reduced by limiting NSAID use to short-acting NSAIDs [34]. Renal effects are also more problematic in seniors, including concerns about the interference of NSAIDs with the efficacy of diuretics.

As in younger patients, opioids have a limited role in treating fibromyalgia in seniors. Opioids require careful monitoring to minimize sedating and cognitive effects, as well as constipation. High-fiber diets, regular exercise, and the use of lactulose and senna are appropriate for minimizing medication-induced constipation.

Summary

- Fibromyalgia affects over 7% of women 60 years old and older.
- Seniors with symptoms suggesting possible fibromyalgia and true muscle weakness should be investigated for other medical conditions.
- Age-appropriate pain assessments in older patients include alternative measures of pain severity, the Geriatric Pain Measure, and the 6-min walking test.

- Fibromyalgia non-medication and medication treatments used in younger patients may require adjustments when used in older patients to account for co-morbid conditions and increased sensitivity to medication side effects.
- Elderly patients are more prone to experience side effects that result in treatment discontinuation.
- Both duloxetine and milnacipran have been shown to be safe and effective when used in older patient populations.
- Pregabalin and gabapentin are excreted by the kidneys, and dosage adjustments will be needed in older patients with renal impairment.
- Regular use of nonsteroidal anti-inflammatory drugs should be limited in older patients with fibromyalgia due to concerns about gastric, cardiovascular, and renal effects.

References

1. Wolfe F, Ross K, Anderson J, Russell IJ, Hebert L. The prevalence and characteristics of fibromyalgia in the general population. Arthritis Rheum. 1995;8:19–28.
2. McNally JD, Matheson DA, Bakowsky VS. The epidemiology of self-reported fibromyalgia in Canada. Chronic Dis Can. 2006;27:9–16.
3. Branco JC, Bannwarth B, Failde I, et al. Prevalence of fibromyalgia: a survey in five European countries. Semin Arthritis Rheum. 2010;39:448–53.
4. Yunus MB, Holt GC, Masi AT, Aldag JC. Fibromyalgia syndrome among the elderly. Comparison with younger patients. J Am Geriatr Soc. 1988;36:987–95.
5. Weiner DK, Sakamoto S, Perea S, Breuer P. Chronic low back pain in older adults: prevalence, reliability, and validity of physical examination findings. J Am Geriatr Soc. 2006;54:11–20.
6. AGS Panel on Chronic Pain in Older Patients. The management of chronic pain in older persons. J Am Ger Soc. 1998;46:635–51.
7. Bruckenthal P, Reid C, Reisner L. Special issues in the management of chronic pain in older adults. Pain Med. 2009;10:S67–78.
8. Herr K, Spratt KF, Garand L, Li L. Evaluation of the Iowa pain thermometer and other selected pain intensity scales in younger and older adult cohorts using controlled clinical pain: a preliminary study. Pain Med. 2007;8:585–600.
9. Ferrell BA, Stein WM, Beck JC. The Geriatric Pain Measure: validity, reliability and factor analysis. J Am Geriatr Soc. 2000;48:1669–73.
10. Enright PL, McBurnie MA, Bittner V, et al. The 6-min walk test: a quick measure of functional status in elderly adults. Chest. 2003;123:387–98.
11. Petrella RJ, Bartha C. Home based exercise therapy for older patients with knee osteoarthritis: a randomized clinical trial. J Rheumatol. 2000;27:2215–21.
12. Song R, Lee EO, Lam P, Bae SC. Effects of tai chi exercise on pain, balance, muscle strength, and perceived difficulties in physical functioning in older women with osteoarthritis: a randomized clinical trial. J Rheumatol. 2003;30:2039–44.
13. Arena JG, Hannah SL, Bruno GM, Meador KJ. Electromyographic biofeedback training for tension headache in the elderly: a prospective study. Biofeedback Self Regul. 1991;16:379–90.
14. Reid MC, Otis J, Barry LC, Kerns RD. Cognitive-behavioral therapy for chronic low back pain in older persons: a preliminary study. Pain Med. 2003;4:223–30.
15. Valkeinen H, Häkkinen A, Hannonen P, Häkkinen K, Alén M. Acute heavy-resistance exercise-induced pain and neuromuscular fatigue in women with fibromyalgia and in healthy controls: effects of strength training. Arthritis Rheum. 2006;54:1334–9.
16. Jones KD, Lipton GL. Exercise interventions in fibromyalgia: clinical applications from the evidence. Rheum Dis Clin N Am. 2009;35:373–91.

17. Stessman J, Hammerman-Rozenberg R, Maaravi Y, Cohen A. Effect of exercise on ease in performing activities of daily living and instrumental activities of daily living from age 70 to 77: the Jerusalem Longitudinal Study. J Am Geriatr Soc. 2002;50:1934–8.
18. Goulding MR. Inappropriate medication prescribing for elderly ambulatory care patients. Arch Intern Med. 2004;164:305–12.
19. Steffens DC, Chung H, Krishnan KR, et al. Antidepressant treatment and worsening white matter on serial cranial magnetic resonance imaging in the elderly: the Cardiovascular Health Study. Stroke. 2008;39:857–62.
20. Stovall R, Brahm NC, Crosby KM. Recurrent episodes of serotonin-reuptake inhibitor-mediated hyponatremia in an elderly patient. Consult Pharm. 2009;24:765–8.
21. Mancini M, Gianni W, Rossi A, Amore M. Duloxetine in the management of elderly patients with major depressive disorder: an analysis of published data. Expert Opin Pharmacother. 2009;10:847–60.
22. Wasan AD, Ossanna MJ, Raskin J, et al. Safety and efficacy of duloxetine in the treatment of diabetic peripheral neuropathic pain in older patients. Curr Drug Saf. 2009;4:22–9.
23. Physician's Desk Reference 2009, edition 63. Cymbalta®. Pages1801–10.
24. Mizukami K, Hatanaka K, Tanaka Y, Sato S, Asada T. Therapeutic effects of the selective serotonin noradrenaline reuptake inhibitor milnacipran on depressive symptoms in patients with Alzheimer's disease. Prog Neuropsychopharmacol Bio Psychiatry. 2009;33:349–52.
25. Rahme E, Dasgupta K, Turecki C, Nedjar H, Galbaud du Fort G. Risks of suicide and poisoning among elderly patients prescribed selective serotonin reuptake inhibitors: a retrospective cohort study. J Clin Psychiatry. 2008;69:349–57.
26. Cappuzzo KA. Treatment of postherpetic neuralgia: focus on pregabalin. Clin Interv Aging. 2009;4:17–23.
27. Physician's Desk Reference 2009, edition 63. Lyrica®. Pages 2527–34.
28. Murphy N, Mockler M, Ryder M, et al. Decompensation of chronic heart failure associated with pregabalin in patients with neuropathic pain. J Card Fail. 2007;13:227–229.
29. Page RL, Cantu M, Lindenfeld J, Hergott LJ, Lowes BD. Possible heart failure exacerbation associated with pregabalin: case discussion and literature review. J Cardiovasc Med (Hagerstown). 2008;9:922–5.
30. Rosenthal NR, Silverfield JC, Wu SC, Jordan D, Kamin M. Tramadol/acetaminophen combination tablets for the treatment of pain associated with osteoarthritis flare in an elderly patient population. J Am Geriatr Soc. 2004;52:374–80.
31. Turajane T, Wongbunnak R, Patcharatrakul T, et al. Gastrointestinal and cardiovascular risk of non-selective NSAIDs and cox-2 inhibitors in elderly patients with knee osteoarthritis. J Med Assoc Thai. 2009;92:S19–26.
32. Johnson AG, Day RO. The problems and pitfalls of NSAID therapy in the elderly (Part I). Drugs Aging. 1991;1:130–43.
33. Scharf S, Kwiatek R, Ugoni A, Christophidis N. NSAIDs and faecal blood loss in elderly patients with osteoarthritis: is plasma half-life relevant? Aust N Z J Med. 1998;28:436–9.
34. Bell GM, Schnitzer TJ. Cox-2 inhibitors and other nonsteroidal anti-inflammatory drugs in the treatment of pain in the elderly. Clin Geriatr Med. 2001;17:489–502.

Gender and Ethnic Issues

Key Chapter Points

- In general, pain sensitivity is greater in women than men.
- Pressure pain threshold at fibromyalgia tender points is significantly lower in women, even in samples where men report more severe fibromyalgia symptoms.
- Men seeking fibromyalgia treatment will typically have more severe symptoms and disability than female treatment seekers.
- Both men and women generally respond similarly to typical fibromyalgia drug and non-drug treatments.
- Ethnicity affects pain tolerance and acceptance of healthcare recommendations.

Keywords Female · Male · Pressure pain threshold · Race

> **Case:** Anil is a 39-year-old whose parents are from India. He is seeking an evaluation for fatigue and severe, chronic widespread pain. "I've had everything poked, prodded, and x-rayed over and over and the doctor never finds anything wrong. My cousin Sumita has fibromyalgia and she said my problems sounded a lot like hers. When I asked the doctor if I could have fibromyalgia he said, 'Probably not. Fibromyalgia is a white woman's disease.' He also pressed all over me on spots he said were fibromyalgia tender point spots. Almost all of the spots hurt, but he said that his fibro patients will usually rate their pain severity to pressing the points around 6 or higher and I rated a number of mine lower than 6. So I guess I can't have fibromyalgia."

Pain experience can be affected by gender and ethnicity. For example, pain threshold and tolerance were evaluated in 64 healthy adults, equally distributed between male and female genders and Middle Eastern vs. Swedish descent [1]. Pain threshold and tolerances to several stimuli were measured, with significant differences noted based

D.A. Marcus, A. Deodhar, *Fibromyalgia*, DOI 10.1007/978-1-4419-1609-9_18,
© Springer Science+Business Media, LLC 2011

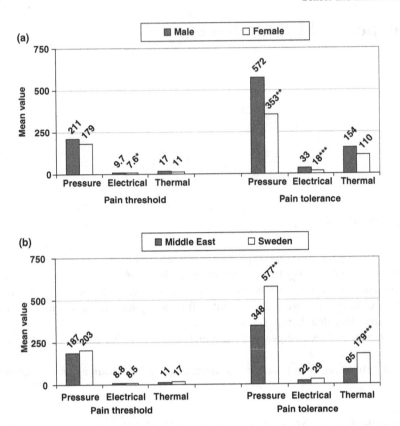

Fig. 1 Gender and ethnic differences in pain in healthy adults (based on Dawson [1]). (**a**) Gender differences, (**b**) ethnic differences. Pressures were evaluated using an algometer and measured in kPa. Electrical pain was measured by current intensity. Thermal pain was assessed by measuring time (seconds) of hand submersion in ice water 0–1°C. Significant differences were seen for gender and ethnicity: $*P < 0.05$, $**P < 0.01$, $***P < 0.001$

on gender and ethnicity (Fig. 1). These data highlight the importance of considering gender and ethnic issues when conducting research studies and caring for patients.

Gender Differences in Fibromyalgia Symptoms and Treatment Response

Pain perception is influenced by gender, with women typically more sensitive to pain than men. Both human and animal experimental studies consistently confirm a lower pain threshold and lower pain tolerance in females compared with males [2–4]. In addition, brain studies using positron emission tomography and functional magnetic resonance imaging reveal objective differences in pain processing between men and women that may explain differences in subjective reporting of the pain experiences [2].

Fibromyalgia Symptoms

Fibromyalgia has consistently been shown to be more prevalent in women, with community samples in North American and Europe reporting fibromyalgia in 2–4% of women vs. < 0.5% of men [2]. Some of this difference in prevalence may be related to gender differences in tender point pain pressure thresholds that might result in an under-diagnosis of fibromyalgia in men. In comparison with healthy men, healthy women have a lower threshold to pressure pain in experiments testing typical fibromyalgia tender point areas for pressure pain threshold [5, 6]. In one study, pressure pain threshold (PPT) over fibromyalgia tender points was compared in female fibromyalgia patients ($N = 20$) and controls ($N = 50$ males and 50 females) [7]. Among controls, PPT was significantly lower in women compared with men (Fig. 2; $P < 0.01$). As expected, PPT was also significantly lower in female fibromyalgia patients compared with controls ($P < 0.0001$). Another study directly evaluated differences in tender point evaluations in fibromyalgia patients that included 40 men and 40 women matched for age and educational level [8]. The

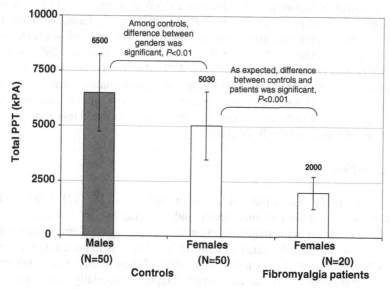

Fig. 2 Pressure pain threshold (PPT) with standard deviation bars in controls and women with fibromyalgia (based on Maquet [7])

number of painful tender points was similar for women and men in this sample (15.4 vs. 15.6). Mean PPT at nine tender sites, however, was significantly lower in women (2.4 vs. 3.6 kg, $P = 0.001$). This difference is particularly interesting since the men in this small study reported significantly more severe fibromyalgia symptoms than the women patients. On a 0–10 Severity Scale, with 10 representing worst status, men in this survey rated pain (8.2 vs. 7.3, $P = 0.029$), fatigue (8.5 vs. 7.2, $P = 0.002$), general well-being (6.8 vs. 6.4, $P = 0.006$), and depression (6.6 vs. 3.8, $P = 0.001$) as significantly worse than their female fibromyalgia counterparts. Irritable bowel syndrome (74% of men vs. 50% of women) and sleep problems (97% vs. 85%) were also significantly more common in these men ($P \leq 0.05$). These studies confirm that males who are healthy and those with fibromyalgia have higher PPT than their female counterparts, even when fibromyalgia symptoms are greater in the men.

Practical pointer

Men generally report lower pain severity to tender point testing.

Gender differences in fibromyalgia patients have not been consistently reported, possibly due to differences in study populations evaluated, such as community vs. clinical samples. While the study cited above reports more severe symptoms in men with fibromyalgia [8], an earlier, larger survey of 536 consecutive fibromyalgia patients (469 women and 67 men) reported similar overall pain severity in women and men (pain severity on a 0–100 scale of 61.2 vs. 59.5, $P = 0.8$) but a significantly higher tender point count (15.6 in females vs. 13.6 in males, $P < 0.001$) and score (37.3 vs. 28.1, $P < 0.001$) in the female patients [9]. Fibromyalgia symptoms occurring more commonly in women in this study included fatigue (91% of females vs. 82% of males, $P < 0.03$), irritable bowel (39% vs. 14%, $P < 0.001$), and generalized pain (67% vs. 49%, $P < 0.001$). In a recent comparison of demographically similar fibromyalgia patients attending tertiary treatment ($N = 33$ men and 33 women), pre-treatment pain severity, affective distress, and general activity were similar between genders, while life interference due to pain was greater for women ($P = 0.005$) [10].

Consultation

Men are less likely to seek medical treatment than women [11, 12], delaying consultation until symptoms become severe and disabling [13, 14]. Therefore, men seen in the clinic for pain complaints often have greater pain severity, interference, and disability than female patients (Table 1) [15, 16]. It is important to recognize that treatment-seekers do not necessarily reflect disease prevalence or symptom reporting that might be seen in community samples, particularly when evaluating men.

Psychological co-morbidity also increases treatment-seeking behavior. Consequently, psychological distress is more commonly seen in fibromyalgia

Table 1 Gender differences in treatment seekers with chronic pain (based on Marcus [16])

Patient characteristic	Men seeking pain treatment (N = 264)	Women seeking pain treatment (N = 452)	P-value
Pain severity (0–100)	71.6	68.2	0.05
Mean days per week with pain	6.4	5.9	< 0.001
Percentage of patients with:			
Constant pain	41.2	26.7	< 0.001
Widespread pain	6.3	6.9	NS
Activities reduced >3 days per week	70.2	56.0	< 0.001
Completely disabled >3 days per week	55.9	37.3	< 0.001
Depression	59.3	58.7	NS
Anxiety	61.6	52.5	NS

NS = not significant

patients than individuals with fibromyalgia surveyed in community samples [17]. A higher prevalence of psychological distress in women in general population samples may therefore also increase the likelihood of seeking treatment among female fibromyalgia patients [18].

Practical pointer

Women are more likely to seek treatment than men. Men who do seek treatment tend to have more severe symptoms and disability than female treatment seekers.

Treatment Response

A recent meta-analysis evaluated treatment outcome in 33 randomized clinical trials utilizing 120 medication and non-medication treatments administered to 7,789 fibromyalgia patients [19]. Treatment outcome was not influenced by gender, suggesting that generally similar responses may be expected for both male and female fibromyalgia patients. Several important gender differences in response to individual treatments, however, have been noted and are described below.

Practical pointer

In general, both men and women respond similarly to typical fibromyalgia drug and non-drug treatments.

Non-medication Treatment Response

Data evaluating gender differences to non-drug analgesic therapies are limited, with a few differences noted for experimental and non-specific chronic pain. Attentional focusing on experimental pain resulted in a 39% reduction in sensory pain score in men, with no reduction of pain in women [20]. Furthermore, gender impact for response to non-medication pain rehabilitation therapies was evaluated in 214 adults with chronic, non-specific spinal pain [21]. Patients were randomized to treatment with behavior-oriented physical therapy, cognitive-behavioral therapy, the combination of both treatments, or usual care and followed for 18 months. Work absence was similarly reduced in women treated with any of the non-drug options, while men treated with cognitive-behavioral therapy alone improved less than those receiving a treatment that included physical therapy. Among fibromyalgia patients attending tertiary treatment ($N = 33$ men and 33 women), both genders responded similarly to pain rehabilitation therapy, although improvement in life interference after treatment was greater in women ($P = 0.02$) [10].

Medication Response

Overall pain relief with analgesics differs between men and women. Men have been found to be more responsive to ibuprofen and μ-opioids (e.g., morphine), while women are more responsive to κ-opioids (e.g., butorphanol) [22–24]. As analgesics have limited efficacy in fibromyalgia in general, these gender differences have only limited impact for fibromyalgia treatment.

Although many treatments can be effectively used for both men and women, duloxetine was shown to be more effective in female fibromyalgia patients, with minimal benefit in males in a double-blind clinical trial in which 184 women and 23 men were treated with duloxetine 60 mg twice daily or placebo [25]. In this study, the female group treated with duloxetine showed significantly better efficacy to all measures tested compared with placebo, while significant benefit was not seen in the small male group for any efficacy measure.

Ethnic Differences in Fibromyalgia Symptoms and Treatment Response

Ethnicity can be defined to include both racial and social influences. Members of an ethnic group may share nationality or cultural heritage, or religious background, while race is typically based on genetically shared physical characteristics. Both race and other ethnic variables may influence an individual's pain experience. While the term ethnicity is sometimes used to describe non-race variables only, race will also be included when using the term ethnicity in this chapter.

Studies consistently report a lower pain tolerance and a greater perception of pain stimuli as unpleasant in African-Americans and Hispanics compared with Caucasians [26–28]. Figure 3 shows experimental pain responses in healthy adults

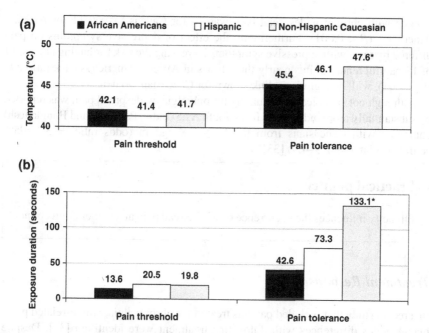

Fig. 3 Differences in pain response based on race (based on Rahim-Williams [29]). (**a**) Heat pain, (**b**) cold pain. Significant differences were seen between African-Americans vs. non-Hispanic Caucasians and Hispanic vs. non-Hispanic Caucasians: *$P < 0.05$

representing three ethnic groups: African-Americans ($N = 63$), Hispanic Americans ($N = 61$), and non-Hispanic Caucasian Americans ($N = 82$) [29]. Heat pain was measured using a heat stimulus that increased by 0.5°C/s. Cold pain was measured by testing duration of exposure to limb immersion in 5°C temperature water. While pain threshold was similar to both stimuli among the three groups, heat and cold pain tolerances were significantly lower in both ethnic groups compared with non-Hispanic Caucasians ($P < 0.05$). Pain tolerances were similar to both stimuli when comparing African-Americans and Hispanics. Reduced pain tolerance to experimental pain in African-Americans supports findings in a population of chronic pain patients that showed similar pain intensity but increased perception of pain unpleasantness in African-Americans compared with Caucasians [30]. Asians similarly demonstrate increased sensitivity to pain [31].

Fibromyalgia Prevalence

Fibromyalgia prevalence was evaluated in a United States community sample of 650 Caucasian and 684 African-American women [32]. Fibromyalgia was diagnosed in 2% of Caucasians and 3% of African-Americans. Median tender point count in women with chronic widespread pain was 14 for Caucasians vs. 11 for African-Americans ($P < 0.001$). Furthermore, the effect of depressive symptoms on pain differed by race, with depressive symptoms increasing the risk for having at least 11 of 18 painful tender points nearly three times in African-Americans (risk ratio 2.8, $P < 0.001$), with no significant link shown for Caucasian women.

Although not specifically evaluating fibromyalgia, widespread pain was reported by substantially more individuals from South Asia (India, Pakistan, and Bangladesh) compared with Caucasians from the United Kingdom (odds ratio = 3.7, 95% confidence interval 2.9–4.9) [33].

Practical pointer

Ethnicity influences the occurrence of widespread pain and tender point count.

Treatment Response

In a recent study that included patients treated for fibromyalgia, ethnic-related pharmacokinetics differences with duloxetine treatment were identified [34]. Despite these differences, the overall steady-state exposure to duloxetine was similar among ethnic groups, suggesting no need to modify duloxetine dosing based on ethnicity.

Race and ethnicity are, however, important to consider when providing educational information about prescribed fibromyalgia therapy. In an interesting, small study, 12 fibromyalgia patients in a rheumatology practice were evaluated [35]. Self-described ethnicity was white in six, black in three, and one each Lebanese, New Zealand British, and Peruvian. Researchers were surprised to uncover that patients who identified themselves as black or another non-white ethnic group reported being suspicious of their doctors and the medications prescribed to them. These results complement those from an earlier study showing that prescribed medications were not purchased by 11% of Caucasians, 16% of Hispanics, and 20% African-Americans [36]. Although there may be a variety of reasons for failure to obtain prescribed medications, which may include cost constraints, misunderstanding or fear about prescribed therapy, or failure of the prescribed therapy to correspond to treatment expectations, these data also support a need for providing additional information and education to help allay patient concerns to improve treatment follow-through.

Practical pointer

Race and ethnicity might influence fibromyalgia patients' acceptance of prescribed therapy.

Summary

- Women in general have a lower pain threshold and tolerance than men.
- Pressure pain threshold over fibromyalgia tender point areas is significantly lower in women than men.
- Gender-related differences in fibromyalgia symptom prevalence and severity have been inconsistent, possibly due to differences in sample selection and the use of patient rather than community samples.
- Men typically seek treatment only when symptom severity and associated disability are substantial.
- In general, medication and non-medication treatments are similarly helpful for reducing fibromyalgia symptoms. A possible exception to this may be duloxetine, which shows more significant benefit in female fibromyalgia patients.
- Pain threshold is affected by ethnicity, with lower thresholds seen in African-Americans and Hispanics.

References

1. Dawson A, List T. Comparison of pain thresholds and pain tolerance levels between Middle Easterners and Swedes and between genders. J Oral Rehabil. 2009;36:271–8.
2. Fillingim RB, King CD, Ribeiro-Dasilva MC, Rahim-Williams B, Riley JL. Sex, gender, and pain: a review of recent clinical and experimental findings. J Pain. 2009;10:447–85.
3. Wiesenfeld-Hallin Z. Sex differences in pain perception. Gend Med. 2005;2:137–45.
4. Vallerand AH, Polomano RC. The relationship of gender to pain. Pain Manag Nurs. 2000; 1:8–15.
5. Chesterton LS, Barlas P, Foster NE, Baxter GD, Wright CC. Gender differences in pressure pain threshold in healthy humans. Pain. 2003;101:259–66.
6. Garcia E, Godoy-Izquierdo D, Godoy JF, Perez M, Lopez-Chicheri I. Gender differences in pressure pain threshold in a repeated measures assessment. Psychol Health Med. 2007;12:567–79.
7. Maquet D, Croisier JL, Demoulin C, Crielaard JM. Pressure pain thresholds of tender point sites in patients with fibromyalgia and in healthy controls. Eur J Pain. 2004;8:111–7.
8. Buskila D, Neumann L, Alhoashle A, Abu-Shakra M. Fibromyalgia syndrome in men. Semin Arthritis Rheum. 2000;30:47–51.
9. Yunus MB, Inanici F, Aldag JC, Mangold RF. Fibromyalgia in men: A comparison of clinical features with women. J Rheumatol. 2000;27:485–90.
10. Hooten WM, Townsend CO, Decker PA. Gender differences among patients with fibromyalgia undergoing multidisciplinary pain rehabilitation. Pain Med. 2007;8:624–32.
11. Linet MS, Celentano DD, Stewart WF. Headache characteristics associated with physician consultation: a population-based survey. Am J Prev Med. 1991;7:40–6.
12. Davies J, McCrae BP, Frank J, et al. Identifying male college students' health needs, barriers to seeking help, and recommendations to help men adopt healthier lifestyles. J Am Coll Health. 2000;48:259–67.
13. Ottesen MM, Kober L, Jorgensen S, Torp-Pedersen C. Determinants of delay between symptoms and hospital admission in 5978 patients with acute myocardial infarction. Eur Heart J. 1996;17:429–37.
14. Johansson E, Long NH, Diwan VK, Winkvist A. Gender and tuberculosis control. Perspectives on health seeking behaviour among men and women in Vietnam. Health Policy. 2000;52:33–51.

15. Marcus DA. Gender differences in treatment-seeking chronic headache sufferers, Headache. 2001;41:698–703.
16. Marcus DA. Gender differences in chronic pain in a treatment-seeking population. J Gend Specif Med. 2003;6:19–24.
17. Aaron LA, Bradley LA, Alarcon GS, et al. Psychiatric diagnoses in patients with fibromyalgia are related to health care-seeking behavior rather than to illness. Arthritis Rheum. 1996;39:436–45.
18. Carroll LJ, Cassidy JD, Cote P. The Saskatchewan Health and Back Pain Survey: the prevalence and factors associated with depressive symptomatology in Saskatchewan adults. Can J Public Health. 2000;91:459–64.
19. Garcia-Campayo J, Magdalena J, Magallón R, et al. A meta-analysis of the efficacy of fibromyalgia treatment according to level of care. Arthritis Res Ther. 2008;10:R81.
20. Keogh E, Hatton K, Ellery D. Avoidance versus focused attention and the perception of pain: differential effects for men and women. Pain. 2000;85:225–30.
21. Jensen IB, Bergstrom G, Ljungquist T, Bodin L, Nygren AL. A randomized controlled component analysis of a behavioral medicine rehabilitation program for chronic spinal pain: are the effects dependent on gender? Pain. 2001;91:65–78.
22. Walker JS, Carmody JJ. Experimental pain in healthy human subjects: gender differences in nociception and in response to ibuprofen. Anesth Analg. 1998;86:1257–62.
23. Gear RW, Miaskowski C, Gordon NC, et al. Kappa-opioid produce significantly greater analgesia in women than in men. Nat Med. 1996;2:1248–50.
24. Miller PL, Ernst AA. Sex differences in analgesia: a randomized trial of mu versus kappa opioid agonists. South Med J. 2004;97:35–41.
25. Arnold LM, Lu Y, Crofford LJ, et al. A double-blind, multicenter trial comparing duloxetine with placebo in the treatment of fibromyalgia patients with or without major depressive disorder. Arthritis Rheum. 2004;50:2974–84.
26. Edwards RR, Fillingim RB. Ethnic differences in thermal pain responses. Psychosomatic Med. 1999;61:346–54.
27. Sheffield D, Biles PL, Orom H, Maixner W, Sheps DS. Race and sex differences in cutaneous pain perception. Psychosom Med. 2000;62:517–23.
28. Edwards RR, Doleys DM, Fillingim RB, Lowery D. Ethnic differences in pain tolerance: clinical implications in a chronic pain population. Psychosom Med. 2001;63:316–23.
29. Rahim-Williams FB, Riley JL, Herrera D, et al. Ethnic identity predicts experimental pain sensitivity in African Americans and Hispanics. Pain. 2007;129:177–84.
30. Riley JL, Wade JB, Myers CD, Sheffield D, Papas RK, Price DD. Racial/ethnic differences in the experience of chronic pain. Pain. 2002;100:291–8.
31. Watson PJ, Latif RK, Rowbotham DJ. Ethnic differences in thermal pain responses: a comparison of South Asian and white British healthy males. Pain. 2005;118:194–200.
32. Gansky SA, Plesh O. Widespread pain and fibromyalgia in a biracial cohort of young women. J Rheumatol. 2007;34:810–7.
33. Palmer B, Macfarlane G, Afzal C, et al. Acculturation and the prevalence of pain amongst South Asian minority ethnic groups in the UK. Rheumatology (Oxford). 2007;46:1009–14.
34. Lobo ED, Quinlan T, O'Brien L, Knadler MP, Heathman M. Population pharmacokinetics of orally administered duloxetine in patients: implications for dosing recommendation. Clin Pharmacokinet. 2009;48:189–97.
35. Lempp HK, Hatch SL, Carville SF, Choy EH. Patients' experiences of living with and receiving treatment for fibromyalgia syndrome: a qualitative study. BMC Musculoskelet Disord. 2009;10:124.
36. Reed M, Hargraves JL. Prescription drug access disparities among working-age Americans. Issue Brief Cent Study Health Syst Change. 2003;73:1–4.

Index